New Paradigms in Healthcare

Series Editors

Maria Giulia Marini, Fondazione ISTUD, Baveno, Italy

Jonathan McFarland, Faculty of Medicine, Autonomous University of Madrid
Madrid, Spain

Editorial Board

June Boyce-Tillman, University of Winchester, North-West University
South Africa and Winchester, UK

Christian Delorenzo, Centre Hospitalier Intercommunal de Créteil
Université Paris-Est Créteil and Créteil, France

Carol-Ann Farkas, MCPHS University, School of Arts and Sciences
Boston, USA

Marco Frey, Scuola Superiore Sant'Anna, Pisa, Italy

Angelika Messner, Christian-Albrechts University, China Centre, Kiel, Germany

Federica Vagnarelli, Danat Clinic, Danat Al Emarat Women's and Children's H
Abu Dhabi, United Arab Emirates

Ourania Varsou, University of Glasgow, College of Medical, Veterinary and Life
Glasgow, UK

Neil Vickers, King's College, Department of English Literature, London, UK

In the first two decades of this new millennium, the self-sufficiency of Evidence-Based Medicine (EBM) have begun to be questioned. The narrative version gradually assumed increasing importance as the need emerged to shift to more biologically, psychologically, socially, and existentially focused models. The terrible experience of the COVID pandemic truly revealed that EBM alone, while being a wonderful scientific philosophy and containing the physician's paternalistic approach, has its limitations: it often ignores both the patient's and physician's perspectives as persons, as human beings; it pays relentless attention to biological markers and not to the more personal, psychological, social, and anthropological ones, removing the emotions, thoughts, and desires of life, focusing on just the "measurable quality" of it.

Health Humanities, Medical Humanities and Narrative Medicine are arts intertwined with sciences that allow to broaden the mindset and approach of healthcare professionals. helping them to produce better care and more well-being.

Aim of this series is to collect "person-centered" contributions, as only a multidisciplinary and collaborative team can meet the challenge of combining the multiple aspects of human health, as well as the health of our planet, and of all the creatures that live on it, in a common effort to stop or reverse the enormous damage committed by humans during our anthropocentric era: a new paradigm of healthcare, education and learning to create a sustainable health system.

Maria Giulia Marini

Non-violent Communication and Narrative Medicine for Promoting Sustainable Health

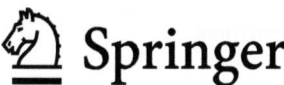

Maria Giulia Marini
Director of ISTUD Sanità e Salute
Milan, Italy

President of EUNAMES – European Narrative Medicine Society
Milan, Italy

ISSN 2731-3247 ISSN 2731-3255 (electronic)
New Paradigms in Healthcare
ISBN 978-3-031-58693-4 ISBN 978-3-031-58691-0 (eBook)
https://doi.org/10.1007/978-3-031-58691-0

© The Editor(s) (if applicable) and The Author(s), under exclusive license to Springer Nature Switzerland AG 2024

This work is subject to copyright. All rights are solely and exclusively licensed by the Publisher, whether the whole or part of the material is concerned, specifically the rights of translation, reprinting, reuse of illustrations, recitation, broadcasting, reproduction on microfilms or in any other physical way, and transmission or information storage and retrieval, electronic adaptation, computer software, or by similar or dissimilar methodology now known or hereafter developed.

The use of general descriptive names, registered names, trademarks, service marks, etc. in this publication does not imply, even in the absence of a specific statement, that such names are exempt from the relevant protective laws and regulations and therefore free for general use.

The publisher, the authors and the editors are safe to assume that the advice and information in this book are believed to be true and accurate at the date of publication. Neither the publisher nor the authors or the editors give a warranty, expressed or implied, with respect to the material contained herein or for any errors or omissions that may have been made. The publisher remains neutral with regard to jurisdictional claims in published maps and institutional affiliations.

This Springer imprint is published by the registered company Springer Nature Switzerland AG
The registered company address is: Gewerbestrasse 11, 6330 Cham, Switzerland

Paper in this product is recyclable.

Foreword

Today, we have no time *for the other.*[1]

This morning, the 12th of October 2023, I woke up and read the news, and the first headline that hit me was, 'Mama, when I die will I go to heaven or hell'. These words were spoken by a 4-year-old Palestinian boy surrounded by the rubble of his home. Quite frankly, I do not understand why I opened my phone to read the news—first mistake of the day.

On another note, my greatest blessing was when the author, Maria Giulia Marini, first asked me to co-edit this series—*New Paradigms in Healthcare,* and secondly invited me to write a short piece for this crucial and timely book. We are living in terrible times; the pandemic lingers but with it subliminal violence that pervades all our lives. Violence takes many forms and shapes and affects different people in diverse ways. Yet, it seems to be absorbed into the twenty-first century life, and one of the main reasons for this phenomenon is that it seems to have no meaning behind the words, or to put it more bluntly, complete lies transformed into words. Communication is the key to what makes us human, how we live our lives, and interact with others. But, if we have no time for 'the other' then we have no time for ourselves, our society, nor our world.

Marini's book is a book that needs to be read, to be pondered on, mulled over, dipped into, and absorbed since it is critical reading for everyone who is concerned about the direction that we are moving. Perhaps, it would be a beneficial and insightful read for our world leaders, but unfortunately, they may not even open it. Marini masterfully weaves together themes from several disciplines, such as poetry, philosophy, and neuroscience. She sheds light on the tragedy of isolation and loneliness, the importance of listening to elder generations and fostering younger ones, and much more.

---

[1] Byung-Chul Han (and Steuer), *Non-Things: Upheaval in the Lifeworld.* Wiley, 2022.

Please read this book and remember that words are the most powerful drug we have, so use them with caution, respect, and without hurting 'the other' because that other is you.

Faculty of Medicine Jonathan McFarland
Universidad Autónoma Madrid
Madrid, Spain

Preface

Violence against healthcare personnel, patients, family members, and citizens is a growing concern that can have severe consequences for both individuals and the healthcare ecosystem, which has been a threat since its inception.

Violence against healthcare personnel refers to any intentional act of aggression, including physical, verbal, or psychological abuse, directed towards individuals working in healthcare roles. This can include doctors, nurses, technicians, and other healthcare workers. Violence against patients refers to the instigation of or performed acts of physical or verbal abuse, including the neglect or denial of their physical, social-emotional, and/or spiritual needs.

The consequences of violence on healthcare personnel can be significant in current situation with a tremendous lack of human resources and infrastructure. It can lead to physical injuries, emotional trauma, and decreased sense of purpose for the work itself. Acts of violence can create a hostile work environment and negatively impact the quality of patient care. Healthcare personnel should be able to perform their duties without fear of harm or intimidation.

Similarly, violence against patients is a serious concern. Patients seek healthcare services with the expectation of receiving care and support, and any form of violence can undermine their trust in the healthcare system. Violence can have long-lasting physical and psychological effects on patients, further exacerbating their fragility and vulnerability.

In healthcare, verbal, or language abuse, refers to using disrespectful, rude, derogatory, or demeaning language towards patients, healthcare personnel, or any individual involved in the healthcare setting. It can occur in various forms such as discriminatory remarks or derogatory language based on race, gender, ethnicity, religion, sexual orientation, or other characteristics.

Patients who experience language violence may feel disrespected, intimidated, or discriminated against, leading to increased anxiety, reluctance to seek care, or diminished satisfaction with the healthcare experience. Healthcare providers encountering language violence may experience emotional distress, decreased job satisfaction, and burnout.

However, violence is also present in stereotypes of our culture, such as the mythization of science, the generalization of adolescents as "rebels," healthism, ageism, the imbalanced power dynamic in many companies and organizations that disadvantage young adults entering the workforce.

Violence, therefore, is also present in the diverging schools of thinking, Evidence-Based Medicine, including Narrative Medicine, which draws from the disciplines of the social and natural sciences and applies the humanities (i.e., philosophy, linguistics, visual and performing arts, and literature) to a healthcare context. It is necessary to find a peaceful and fruitful alchemy for using both Science and Humanities, stopping any dichotomic opposition, and increasing the competence and knowledge of Narrative Medicine.

Narrative Medicine is an approach that emphasizes the importance of storytelling and patient narratives in healthcare. It recognizes that illness and healthcare experiences are not just medical conditions but also personal and subjective experiences.

By listening to and understanding patients' stories, healthcare providers can gain insight into their experiences, emotions, and values. This understanding can help healthcare providers develop more patient-centered care plans, improve patient satisfaction, and enhance overall healthcare outcomes. Narrative Medicine can also help healthcare providers cope with the emotional demands of their work and maintain empathy towards patients.

Nonviolent communication is an extraordinary skill to develop to transform conversations from brutal and dangerous to peaceful and safe spaces. The method is based on fact-checking, discovery of emotions, explication of needs, and definition of action.

This book is rich in quotes and metaphors from literature, philosophy, and neuroscience. The learning will also be related to analogical thinking, a cognitive approach to learning and problem-solving that involves drawing parallels and connecting different concepts or domains.

Analog thinking recognizes that many concepts or problems in one domain can be related to or understood through concepts or problems in another, thus enabling one to solve complex problems through familiar scenarios. Analog thinking helps promote creativity, critical thinking, and problem-solving skills by encouraging individuals to look beneath the surface and find connections between seemingly unrelated concepts or domains. It allows for a more holistic understanding of the subject matter and facilitates the application of knowledge in novel situations. Health Humanities can be used in scientific and clinical contexts to develop empathy, compassion, creativity, and sound decision-making skills. These four skills are in critical demand in healthcare organizations.

The pursuit of strategies to prevent and respond to violence using the heritage of Health Humanities can create safer, more empathetic, compassionate, and lighter healthcare environments. More than this, at congresses, Sciences, Medicine, and Humanities can talk with no hidden or explicit violence, as is far too often witnessed among each other, since every topic will enrich the quality of caring, curing and healing, and in the grand scheme of things, this living health ecosystem.

Milan, Italy   Maria Giulia Marini

Acknowledgments

My experience in the healthcare area covers most of my life; throughout these years, I have met so many kind and enlightened healthcare and social workers, who have spent their entire lives caring for and curing their patients or people seeking aid. I'm so grateful for what I have learned from them: caring, responsibility, competence, positive attitude. However, I have also met healthcare professionals, who despite being exceptional at adhering to standard protocols and procedures, discouraged their patients from asking questions and sharing their experience of living with an illness. Some clinicians feel narrative medicine as an intrusion on their common practice managing their visit, very much related to the target organ they visit, and to nothing else. Doing narrative medicine is an act of curiosity, courage, and deepening relationships within the healthcare ecosystem, to create reciprocity among those in this setting, even in an unpleasant situation, whereas the mere acts of writing a prescription and following protocols cannot alone bring quality of care.

When I started to write this book about nonviolent communication and narrative medicine, I saw that a multitude of patients and vulnerable people felt as though they could not freely speak, or decide their own future, and even if they had such an opportunity, they doubted that their perspective would be considered because their perception, based on some doctors' view, is totally unreliable. However, these sentiments ring true also for a multitude of doctors, nurses, and carers who would like to add narrativity to their practice which harvests better relationships between all those in the healthcare setting. Hyper-bureaucracy within the healthcare system is a risk factor for erasing the human side of doctors, nurses, aid professionals, and even patients.

Keeping the people in silence is a form of violence, deciding for others what's best for their health is another form of violence, and boasting within the scientific community that one "kind" of research approach is better than another, without trying to have a constructive conversation, is another form of violence.

Most importantly, I'm grateful that my professional life has given me the chance to bear witness to the polarization of viewpoints in healthcare regarding the integration of the humanities to research and medical practice, which would give leeway to the human need to narrate feelings, wishes, thoughts, before, during, and after the onset of the malady. It has been my experience that the denial of giving importance to these human aspects is an injustice and cruelty.

At ISTUD, I learned that the ethnographic approach enriched my scientific background with the genuine need to draw meaning from suffering, which can be reached through narrativity. I learned to honor the stories told by people, groups, and organizations. Because of utilizing an ethnographic research approach, together with the use of art therapy, I was compelled to study linguistics over the last 8 years. I'm grateful to the linguists of Griffith University at Brisbane, including Cliff Goddard; to Anna Wierzbicka at the Australian National University for encouraging the interplay between linguistics and narrative medicine. I'd also like to thank Bert Peeters, an extraordinary mentor in linguistics—you will be always in my heart.

So many people thank me, people who, when they knew I was writing a book linking nonviolence to narrative medicine, encouraged me by affirming the need for this book. Yes, while I'm writing these lines Europe is facing a war and another has just begun in Israel. But still, on this dystopian planet, I indulge speaking about kindness, conversations, and listening, among generations, carers and patients, colleagues, and among sciences. Maybe I'm a utopian, but I think that this is one of the reasons why I was given life.

The words used by trendsetters now are "activism," "sustainability," and "Evidence-based Medicine." I would love that "Awareness," "Responsibility," and "Linguistic-based Care" could become more used and known.

Some of the people I'm grateful for have come and gone, others still alive, yet among them are philosophers, scientists (especially neuroscientists), doctors, nurses, artists, authors, poets, anonymous and known patients.

The names I wish to share are my son, Gabriele, a political philosopher who inspired me to clarify the boundary between the individuals (selfish) and their community (altruism), in organizations, afterwards with my adaption to the healthcare system; the dearest friends of EUNAMES (the European Narrative Medicine Society): June Boyce-Tillmann, Susana Magalhaes, Teresa Casal, Mariel Vespa, Francesca Bracco, Enrica Leydi, Ourania Varsou, John Launer, Neil Vickers, Muiris Houston, Jonathan Mc Farland, Christos Lionis, and all the other participants; the colleagues at ISTUD of the past and the present time: Luigi Reale, Paola Chesi, Alessandra Fiorencis, Antonietta Cappuccio, Francesco Minetti, Roberta Invernizzi, Roberta Termini, Francesca Bracco, Francesca Frigo. To Claudio Mencacci, Maurizio Pompili, Salvatore Varia, Matteo Balestreri, and Ubaldo Sagripanti, I give my appreciation for the "Fuori dal Blu" narrative research project on people with depression.

I'd like to give a special thanks to Erika Greco for helping in structuring chapters, and to Celeste Ortiz, a fabulous, talented student at Northwestern University who brought fresh insights and reviewed this manuscript improving my English—all my gratitude!

And to the participants of Masters in Applied Narrative Medicine who enriched this book bringing their own narratives collection: Giovanna Borriello, Alessandra Cecconello, Angela Micheli, Filippo Arrigoni, Giorgio Bardellini, and their fantastic colleagues. Also, to Marco Trabucchi and Arianna Romano for the REMIND project on Alzheimer, and Alessandro Re, who was engaged in the narrative research on doping in youth athletes.

To my family, to my mother Giulia who instilled in me the love for philosophy and arts, to my father Antonio, who instilled me the passion for science and therapy; to my sister Marina, and her daughter Evelyn, who is learning to read fast and will be a wonderful carer, and to my soul sister Letizia, a wonderful carer. And again to, to my son Gabriele who has opened wis wings and learnt to fly, and to his father and my dearest friend, Enzo, who, as a social worker, helped me to see the need to construct a bridge between science, clinic, and society; and as a yoga expert, avid cook, and dancer, has been teaching me how to enjoy life.

Contents

1	**Nonviolent Communication in Health Care: Learning from "The Tempest"**	1
	1.1 Prologue	1
	1.2 Epilogue	2
	1.3 Violence	3
	1.4 Violence in the Vernacular Language	6
	1.4.1 Non-violent Communication	7
	1.5 Epilogue: Prosperous Unveiled	9
	1.6 Practice Time	12
	References	13
2	**How Many Narrative Medicines Are in the History of Human Beings?**	15
	2.1 Language, the History of Its Use	15
	2.2 Between Factual and Symbolic Language in Healthcare	17
	2.3 Can Communication Alone Be More Effective Than Treatment Alone?	18
	2.3.1 How Many "Narrative Medicines"? Helping Ourselves with the Name of the Rose	20
	2.4 Practice Time	22
	References	23
3	**Communicating Science to Citizens, Patients, and Doctors: The Violence of Becoming Dogmatic**	25
	3.1 "Science Says So"	26
	3.2 The Blaming Culture and Hesitancy Towards Vaccination	30
	3.3 From the Violence of Social Pressure to the Finding of a Common "Good"	31
	3.4 Practice Time	32
	References	33

4	**The Violence of the Loss and Lack of Rituals**	35
	4.1 The Funeral Rituals	40
	4.2 Practice Time	43
	4.2.1 Losing a Patient for a Surgeon [5]	43
	4.2.2 The Loss of a Patient from the Perspective of a Nurse [8]	46
	References...	47

5	**Communication in Case of Isolation: The Tribute to the Young People, Distance Learning, Hikikomori and Anorexia Cases**..	49
	5.1 The Violence of Social Pressure	51
	5.1.1 The Forced Hikikomori Youth Lockdown	52
	5.1.2 To Eat or Not to Eat, This Is the Problem	57
	5.2 Invitation to Live	60
	5.3 Practice Time	61
	References...	64

6	**Nonviolent Communication with the Older People, Honoring Them During Their Last Years, and The Violence of Agism**........	65
	6.1 The Threshold of Elderly Today	66
	6.2 The Witnessing of Living with Elders with Alzheimer	67
	6.3 The Isolation Damages	69
	6.3.1 Agism, A Short-Sighted Prejudice.....................	70
	6.4 Narrative Medicine with Elderly in Nursing Home..............	71
	6.5 The Natural Threshold.....................................	72
	6.6 Practice Time	73
	References...	76

7	**Where We Were and Are Now with Digital Health in Communication**...	77
	7.1 Robot	79
	7.2 Towards Alienation	82
	7.3 Developing a Wise Telemedicine............................	83
	7.4 The Naissance of a New Paradigm: Chat GPT	85
	7.5 Chat GPT in the Healthcare System	86
	7.6 Practice Time	87
	7.6.1 The Case of Technology Replacing Doctors' Human Actions in Diagnosis and Intervention..................	87
	7.6.2 The Doctor-Engineer Emerging Role	89
	References...	90

8	**Violence of Power in the Role Status, Time and Size: Finding the Right Words, Timing and Dimension**	93
	8.1 The Risk of Narcissistic Disorder in Health Care Provider.......	94
	8.1.1 Dr. King of Hearts	95
	8.2 No Time to Say "Hello"...................................	97

	8.3	Tea-Time and The Rabbit Hole	99
	8.4	Practice Time	100
		8.4.1 Reading of Patients' Violence Against Health Care Providers. Expanding Our Point of View	100
		8.4.2 Reading the Narrative on Violence Written By a Doctor Who Prefers to Remain Anonymous	102
		8.4.3 Learning What is Empathy from a Neuroscientific Point of View	105
		8.4.4 Mastering Style of Communication	107
		8.4.5 Finding Time to Say Hallo to Alice	107
	References		108
9	**The Ceaseless Cycle of Violence, Cause of Malaise and Cooperation of Human Beings as Cause of Well Being**		109
	9.1	The Historical Era of the Anthropocene	109
		9.1.1 What Health, What Rights?	113
	9.2	Human Rights	114
	9.3	Rights for Disabled People	118
	9.4	Children, The Future Generations	124
		9.4.1 The Rights of Children and Adolescents	124
		9.4.2 Illness of Children and Play	126
	9.5	The Courses and Resources	127
	9.6	Courses and Recurrences	128
	9.7	Practice Time	129
		9.7.1 Green Pass Between Utopic and Dystopic	129
		9.7.2 Right to Play to Lightness for Children, Adults, and Older People	133
		9.7.3 Playfulness	133
		9.7.4 Alignment or Misalignment for a More Sustainable Ecosystem	135
	References		139
10	**Multiple Intelligences to A Healthcare Wonderland**		141
	10.1	How Do We Define Intelligence?	141
		10.1.1 *The Queen's Gambit*: Beth Harmon	142
		10.1.2 The Voluntas	145
		10.1.3 Self-realization: The Reason for Living	146
		10.1.4 Recognition	147
		10.1.5 Smart Healthcare Providers	148
		10.1.6 Healthcare Wonderland	150
	10.2	Practice Time of This Last Chapter	151
		10.2.1 The Listening Scale	151
		10.2.2 Nesting Multiple Intelligence with Not Violent Communication	153
		10.2.3 Moving from Violence to Peace	155
	References		158

About the Author

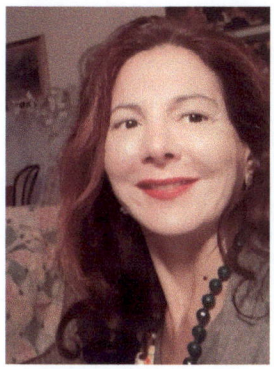

Maria Giulia Marini is an epidemiologist and counsellor, currently working as the Scientific and Innovation Director of the Health Care Area at ISTUD.

She has more than 35 years of professional experience in the healthcare sector, having worked in organizational and social consulting and training in healthcare. She teaches Narrative Medicine and Medical Humanities at several national and international universities, such as the University La Sapienza in Rome. Marini has developed an innovative scientific methodology to perform narrative medicine. In 2016, she became a Reviewer for the World Health Organization for narrative methods in Public Health. She is the author of the volume *Narrative Medicine: Bridging the Gap Between Evidence-Based Care and Medical Humanities* for Springer, translated in Italian and Chinese, *The languages of care in narrative medicine*, as well as a number of international publications on Narrative Medicine in 2018. She published the item Narrative Medicine for the Encyclopaedia Treccani in 2020 and the item Empathy in the Neuroscience chapter for Treccani. She is the editor of the bilingual (Italian and English) online journal Chronicles of Health and Narrative Medicine. She has been the Founder and she is the current President of the European Narrative Medicine Society (EUNAMES) since 2020, and in 2021, began editing a new series titled *New Paradigms in Health Care*.

She is a speaker in national and international academic and institutional contexts. Finally, *the pursuit of knowledge, intelligent kindness*, and *activism* are her three keywords.

Chapter 1
Nonviolent Communication in Health Care: Learning from "The Tempest"

1.1 Prologue

PROSPERO
Now, does my project gather to a head:
My charms crack not; my spirits obey; and time
Goes upright with his carriage. How's the day?
ARIEL
On the sixth hour, at which time, my lord,
You said our work should cease.
PROSPERO
I did say so when first I raised the Tempest. Say, my spirit,
How fares the King and's followers?
ARIEL
Confined together in the same fashion as you gave in charge,
Just as you left them, all prisoners, sir,
In the line grove which weather-fends your cell.
They cannot budge till your release. The king,
His brother and yours abide all three distracted,
Your charm so strongly works,
That if you now beheld them, your affections
It would become tender.
PROSPERO
Dost thou think so, spirit?
ARIEL
Mine would, sir, were I human.
PROSPERO
And mine shall.
Hast thou, which art but air, a touch, a feeling

© The Author(s), under exclusive license to Springer Nature
Switzerland AG 2024
M. G. Marini, *Non-violent Communication and Narrative Medicine for Promoting Sustainable Health*, New Paradigms in Healthcare,
https://doi.org/10.1007/978-3-031-58691-0_1

Of their afflictions, and shall not myself,
One of their kind, that relish all as sharply,
Passion as they, be kindlier moved than thou art?
Though with their high wrongs, I am struck to the quick,
Yet with my nobler reason 'gaitist my fury. Do I take part? The rarer action is
In virtue than in vengeance: they being penitent,
The sole drift of my purpose doth extend. Not a frown further.
Go release them, Ariel:
My charms I'll break, their senses I'll restore,
And they shall be themselves.
ARIEL
I'll fetch them, sir.
Exit
PROSPERO
But this rough magic
I here abjure, and, when I have required
Some heavenly music, which even now I do,
To work mine end upon their senses that
This airy charm is for, I'll break my staff,
Bury it certain fathoms in the earth,
And deeper than did ever plummet sound
I'll drown my book.

1.2   Epilogue

SPOKEN BY PROSPERO
Now my charms are all overthrown,
And what strength I have's mine own,
Which is the most faint
But release me from my bands
With the help of your good hands:
Gentle breath of yours, my sails
Must fill, or else my project fails,
Which was to please. Now I want
Spirits to enforce, art to enchant,
And my ending is despair,
Unless I be relieved by prayer,
Which pierces so that it assaults
Mercy itself and frees all faults.
As you from crimes would pardoned be,
Let your indulgence set me free [1]

With this extraordinary monologue about forgiveness and liberation, after a life of abuse suffered, exiled from his land, the Duchy of Milan, Prospero breaks the magic art he learned to wield on the island which helped him to do justice, absolves his executioners, frees the spirit of Nature and of Good (Ariel) and Evil (Caliban, who, ironically, promises to behave righteously and honestly) and asks for indulgence from us, the reading and viewing public.

I wanted to write about Nonviolent Communication [2] in healthcare, using, not only actual cases and facts, but also narrative, fiction through the analogue method [3] (borrowed from Health Humanities), and especially this powerful excerpt of literature drawn from "The Tempest" by William Shakespeare. So before entering the desired transition from Violent to Nonviolent communication, let's shed light on the analogue method, which will be a filrouge all over the pages of this book.

Analogical thinking, at the basis of the analogue method, is the implementation of a process of recognizing similarities between objects and relationships that connect them placed in different situations, often referring to even distant experiential contexts. In the case where this recognition process takes place, the situations seem to be similar. What emerges as the effect of the recognition of an analogy is the objectification of a kind of identity of the relationships between the objects in the two situations, with the zeroing of differences between the characters of the objects themselves. The power of analogical thinking lies in its ability to activate the transfer of relationships and properties from within a given experiential context to another, lesser known one the moment the latter is recognized as resembling/analogous to the former. In our specific case, the moving act from "The Tempest" starts as a tragedy full of violence, and it ends up as a Comedy with a happy ending in the paradigm of Nonviolent Communication. First, we must analyse, before the end, the possible meaning of violence.

1.3 Violence

Violence is a "strong" word that cannot be easily replaced by others. From the Oxford definition of Violence:

The exercise of physical force to inflict injury on, or cause damage to, persons or property; action or conduct characterized by this treatment or usage tending to cause bodily injury or forcibly interfere with personal freedom.

The etymon of the word violence comes from a composition of two Latin words, "Vis" and "Opulentus." The former means literally strength and violence, and the latter—Opulentus—is exaggerated, powerful, or virulent. Therefore, Strength, combined with the word Power, can be summed up to create the word violence.

Curious is the etymon of violence in ancient Greece; she is a minor goddess, "Bia," and the sister of Nike, meaning victory (as the Nike brand), and Cratos, from which every kind of word which ends in—cracy, such as democracy, plutocracy, technocracy, originates.

The World Health Organization [4] defines violence as "the intentional use of physical force or power, threatened or actual, against oneself, another person, or against a group or community, which either results in or has a high likelihood of resulting in injury, death, psychological harm, maldevelopment, or deprivation." In this case, the WHO focuses solely on violent human behaviours, neglecting that violence may be found in nature as well.

According to the Natural Semantic Metalanguage [5] (NSM), a theory that attempts to reduce the semantics of all lexicons down to a restricted set of 65 semantic primitive universals, which have the exact translation in every language. The primes are ordered together to form explications, we could try to get to the core of the word violence using grammar and words drawn from the NSM:

Violence is when:
I want you (and the others) to do this;
Maybe you don't want it;
Maybe the thing I want you to do makes you feel bad;
Maybe I want to do something bad on (your) body
Maybe I want to say bad words that make you feel bad
Maybe I do not know that all these things are bad for you (and the others)
Maybe I know that all these things are bad for you and good for me.

When we use the NSM, we see a sharp distinction between the first-person speaker, and the other (s): *I, You, Others, and People*—words of the NSM- are very well distinguished: missing in this universal dictionary is the "we", the "us", showing that these pronouns are not even considered in every cultural society around the world, but this concept, and its mirroring word has to be built with time and trust.

However, we can expand our horizons. Violence is not just a result of human deeds but can be found almost everywhere, even in natural events and laws. For example, the change of health status, in some cases moving quickly and abruptly, while in other cases, with slower paces towards the disease. What about the possible violence of labour pains? And the difficult age of adolescence? And the getting older? And death?

A sudden outbreak, a slower cognitive impairment, are at the edge of possible violence when we experience a loss in health according to the biological, psychological, social, and existential model: the "quiddity" in the middle of the line can be mastered and coped with, but they are generally undesired events. Therefore, in the "Violence of nature", with its biological rules, we need to take refuge in a safe and trustworthy space and keep violence out of the door.

In medicine, violent communication is often hidden behind ritual words, gestures, bureaucratic actions, and organisational culture. Regarding this last one, which is the reference frame, violence is the continuous shortage of resources in healthcare practice; it is the fast discharge for economic reasons when a patient has not recovered yet; it is the abolishment of convalescence, short-term contracts, inadequate salaries for hospital staff, unreasonably long shifts for the providers, never-ending waiting lists, and frustratingly short visits. These are the leading organisational features that indicate a deterioration of the national and international health services.

We observe violent communication in a patient's narrative which satirically describes the physician persona; they mention the ritual "take off your clothes", "now give me your arm", and "don't be scared, it is only a little needle". The jargon in the medical field is typically either technical or hierarchic since the organisational

1.3 Violence

culture is one of having two possible "chiefs". The former is the cliché "patronizing" doctor who decides for you, not with a gentle nudge, but with a commanding countenance. This kind of doctor tells you exactly which drugs to take, without taking the time to obtain a full picture of the patient's life. The latter is completely stuck in the domain of Evidence-Based Medicine where numbers orient the decision-making, doctors are its ambassadors, and they are considered the most reliable today. However, if the culture promoting this method of data collection, of truth-seeking, were the best method, we should not have such a low rate of adhesions to treatments.

Let's explore the iCount [6] study on diabetes:

> The iCount study was set up as an offshoot of the TODAY2 study, which showed that young people with an early diagnosis of type 2 diabetes appear to be rapidly accumulating complications, including dyslipidemia, hypertension, broader cardiovascular disease, kidney disease, retinopathy, and poor pregnancy outcomes.
> For their longitudinal study, Trief and colleagues measured medication adherence in 381 young people (mean age 26 years) with type 2 diabetes, of whom 212 were taking oral antidiabetic medications, and 192 were being treated with insulin.
> At study enrollment, an extensive and validated psychosocial assessment was carried out for all participants, assessing factors such as attitudes toward Diabetes, treatment beliefs, self-management efficacy, diabetes distress, depression, anxiety, and level of treatment support. The cohort was followed up over time, and a broad assessment of adherence based on a cutoff was made one year later.
> During the year, regular assessments such as unannounced phone pill counts were made on a 3-monthly basis for the oral medication group. In the insulin group, adherence data were collected by self-report.
> Of 171 patients in the oral medication group assessed at 12 months, 112 had low treatment adherence, defined as less than 80%, at baseline. Factors increasing this likelihood included having more concerns about antidiabetic medications since they could cause harm, the possibility for overuse, and insecurities over healthcare coverage, with odds ratios (ORs) of 1.4 and 4.9, respectively.
> Over the year, mean adherence rates declined from 57.9% at baseline to 51.4% in those taking oral medications. Factors significantly predicting low adherence at 12 months included housing insecurity, having at least two material insecurities, and believing that antidiabetic medications are harmful or overused. Once baseline adherence had been considered, only housing insecurity and reporting at least two material insecurities remained significant risk factors.

> In the group treated with insulin (157 assessed at 12 months), 57 had low adherence at baseline. These individuals were significantly more likely to believe that medications are overused (OR = 1.9) and harmful (OR = 2.4), feel less supported in the self-management of their condition (OR = 0.5), and report at least one material insecurity (OR = 2.9).
> The same factors predicting low adherence at baseline predicted low adherence at 12 months, with the addition of higher diabetes distress and food insecurities. After considering adherence at baseline, only beliefs about medications being harmful or overused remained significant.
> Good social determinants, such as home, income, and a decent environment, were crucial factors for concordance to therapy, and, when achieved, patients were less sceptical against drugs compared to people living in vulnerable conditions. However, independently from their cultural context, the authors conclude that instead of using prescriptive jargon, they could have asked questions such as "Please tell me what you think about taking the medicines that I have recommended. What concerns do you have?"
>
> If we read the whole study asking ourselves, "Are we asking the right questions to patients?" we understand that we are dealing with very empathic doctors, eager to know patient's life conditions beyond the disease. We should remember that trust is a virtue that matures over time, and it should not be taken for granted. In the doctors' patients' encounter, there is an initial struggle, a tension [7], embedded in this kind of relationship, very asymmetric in terms of power.

This example on Diabetes is a good opening model on how to carry out research that does not only focus on clinical symptoms but also health drivers according to the possible determinants of WHO as (1) access to care, (2) reimbursement of the visits, (3) having a job, income, house, etc. This is an exemplary model of how an EBM study could be designed considering social issues.

1.4 Violence in the Vernacular Language

Let me bring a light and short example: while writing these lines, I suffer from the Omicron-5 Covid disease—nothing serious but, indeed, more than a simple flu. So far, my sore throat is the worst I have experienced, and I have difficulty eating. People around me with phone calls (and I do not have a voice now) or messages in the majority are divided into two categories: some who use the imperative tense: "You have to get better," "Take care of yourself," and "heal soon" "get back in shape up" or, in the kindest situation, "try to recover."

I know there is affection behind these words, but they are probably among the most used words by doctors and caregivers. Well, even if their intentions are good, these people are violent and short-sighted because they do not consider the limits of each human being. Is there a magic recipe to recover fast from COVID-19? Some others, however, mainly doctors, wish me a nice recovery; without that, "I feel ashamed if this good recovery does not come." Each verb conjugated with the imperative tense acts as a wall or barrier because it does not open to really understanding what the other person is experiencing, it prioritises the needs of the self, and hence, is a way to block conversation. If one must use the imperative form to emerge from the fist of violence, we must specify, with facts, the reason of this order. Remember that an order, as a prescription, is a top-down event, not a peer-to-peer relationship. We should ask ourselves: What kind of relationship do we wish to nourish with our patients, colleagues, and friends? Would we like to hear and learn from their feelings and needs?

But there are much worse instances like in the case of my old friend who is part of a WhatsApp group chat I am in. One evening, she writes that she cannot attend a proposed annual dinner since she was readmitted to the hospital to treat her breast cancer metastasis. Most of the people in the chat were very nice, writing, "We will wait for you" and "We are close to you", to show support and friendship. Suddenly, one person wrote, "What the hell are you doing? Heal and get out of the hospital". The chat was "frozen"-- nobody dared to write anything else but contacted this woman separately.

I insist that using the imperative mode with patients is an act of violence, especially if we cannot counterbalance our words with a welcoming body language made of tenderness and sympathy. Now it is time to unveil what is nonviolent communication and its technique.

1.4.1 Non-violent Communication

Nonviolent Communication (NVC) is a communication approach based on principles of nonviolence. It is not a technique to end disagreements but rather a method designed to increase empathy and improve the quality of life of those who utilize the method and the people around them. It is an old technique developed by Marshall Rosenberg, an American psychologist, in second half of last century; quite resembling Rogers's point of view of a person-cantered program, it became more popular under the name of compassion communication or empathetic communication, with the word "Violence" possibly often upgrade new semantic formulas. The NVC found many applications in health care, education, diplomacy, family therapy, and working organization, but broader in self-development.

> Here are the steps for nonviolent communication for a patient-centred approach:
>
> 1. Observations: a deep reality check, according not only to the biomedical model but also to the biological, psychological, social, and existential model. How do we fact-check? Asking questions, willing to be informed before expressing any possible evaluation about the deeds.

2. Feelings: cognitive empathy to catch those emotions and to create a safe space. How to do this? By acknowledging the feelings of others and about oneself in the relationship. But first come the others, and here, asking the questions about, "How do you feel because of...?" Not simply "How do you feel," since it is a too vague question. We are not used to giving the nuances to our emotions, and we could try not to use only the five primary emotions as sadness, anger, shame, joy, and fear, but be more accurate about this. For instance, fear; Is it anxiety? Is it panic? Is it terror? Is it something that has not found a name but can be well expressed through a metaphor?
3. Needs, it means creating the environment so that the person can express his /her own needs without fearing judgment and without being submitted to rules that may not be followed in the future. The needs are, of course, related to the analysis of emotions. According to Rosenberg, it is impossible to separate the emotions of human beings from the needs.
4. Requests: the possibility to open and express oneself independently by the asymmetric knowledge position of the doctor and the patient: the doctor is competent, but so is the patient. According to Rosenberg, the request should be expressed with the words "I want to..." and not "I don't want to...". This is because we are more focused on avoiding risks and malevolent experiences than wishing to enjoy life as we can despite this being "a wild world."

Nonviolent communication also helps in maintaining a good quality of life and a civil way of professional life within the organization through authentic self-expression, including spirituality, a topic that is often deemed personal and private. Focusing more on needs rather than the "obsolete" idea of being right or wrong brings peace and harmony, even in the frantic working environment. Moreover, it helps focus, affiliation, trust, it preserves from abuse of power and brutalities. *Per absurdum*, violent communication is when we use relationships only to manipulate others, imposing our vision of the world with little white lies. Persuasion might lead to propaganda, even in the medical field. For instance, propaganda pro-vaccination and against vaccination for Sars-Covid (we will explore this issue in the chapter "Faith in Science," but it is worth mentioning how the propaganda was polarized and exploded in riots in the street) [8].

An example from "daily life in a friendship between two people: one complains of being neglected by the other, of course perception plays a role, but it can be a biased perception." Fact-checking observation dictates that one goes to WhatsApp to count the messages, the occasions of encounters generated by one and the other, but more, the quality of the messages the thought behind each sending. Sometimes, there is confirmation that one has been overlooked; sometimes, one discovers opposite realities. This is also true when analysing the facts between doctors and patients, so nonviolent communication is not a simple technique of "the politically correct philosophy', but encompasses health and illness, being neglected, or being cured. However, knowing the limits of this polarization

1.5 Epilogue: Prosperous Unveiled

We return to "the Tempest" for a final examination; nonviolent communication does not mean being Zen, letting everything go, taking things easy, not even 'turning the other cheek.' It is, learning from Prospero, the Duke of Milan, to help oneself with the magic arts of words to do oneself justice to express the right to live; it means to metaphorically undermine – the reasons, – and the continual contradiction of the other. For this reason, when Prospero restores sensibility to those who usurped him in the role, he gives nothing but a new awareness in his unravelling, which comes, however, slowly; 'Their intelligence begins to mount', like the tide. But very slowly we discover that Prospero is our teacher, some will understand him, and others will watch the performance without grasping the main meaning of the comedy.

It takes time and patience to become "good listeners," consider how at first the "usurpers" were un-sentient, and only after the shipwreck, having lost all their reference and having been at the mercy of the elements, were they then able to understand the damage done. after Prospero who is ahead of everyone in reason and awareness.

The first phase of not violent communication are the observed facts and here in "The Tempest", the main actors: with what happened and what did not happen. And the deeds were made of violence: Prospero was betrayed, defrauded of his kingdom, thrown onto an island with his daughter, resorting to seeking revenge by causing a storm that would shipwreck his traitors and their relatives on that very land. Tired of violent revenge, he decides to appease himself and grant forgiveness.

With his fact-checking attitude, Prospero cannot pretend that he has not been despoiled of his kingdom and that Caliban almost raped his daughter Miranda. The facts are there, on the table, and in the words. What then works the 'miracle of change' is when the raw truth, including the truth existing in dreams, 'of which we are made of the same stuff' comes out. Time, the suspension of judgement on both sides, reflection, another space-time dimension. Evidently, it is not the use of the indicative mode, but in contrast, the subjunctive mode-- the world of nostalgia and desire, and of the optative mode. The optative form is a Greek invention, that was born to express desires, dreams, and wishes. In The Tempest, Prospero creates bonds and imprisons every living being, including spirits, until his final decision to liberate this island, his new kingdom: it is an island of pause, far from the historical events that are in the meantime turning Europe upside down; we do not even know topographically where this unknown island is.

Yet it is not John Donne's Island, 'no man is an island', which refers to Europe [9]. It is a world inhabited by all the characters necessary to develop the story, including the forces of nature, that will bring Prospero to the final confrontation and consequent forgiveness, considering that nobody will give him back the twelve years he spent away from the Duchy of Milan. And that's a thorough fact-checking, according to NVC.

The second step of nonviolent communication is 'the expression of one's emotions, of one's state of being: "That, if you saw them now, you would have tenderness of them. Says Ariel, and Prospero replies, do you think so, spirit?" And Ariel: "I would if I were human," And the magician: *"Then I will be. Thou who art but air, thou art as if touched with a sense, A sorrow for their afflictions, And I, who am of the same kind, who suffer the same passions, Shall I not, man, Move more than thou? Deeply with their blows, they have lacerated me, but against my fury, I side with the noblest reason. The works of virtue are rarer..."* Ariel and Prospero communicate with each other in a nonviolent way: they listened deeply to each other's words, and they ask each other questions to make sure they have understood beyond their emotions. Going further, they make explicit, as in the third point of nonviolent communication, their needs respecting each other; Ariel is made of air and wants freedom, meanwhile, Prospero desires a return to his homeland. The dialogue between them is easy, not guilt-ridden, but rather reflective; there is no anger in Prospero's words nor rancour in those of Ariel, who has faithfully served the magician all this time. After explicating one's needs, the consequence of this lightness between the parties is the final request. Thus, Ariel asks for freedom and Prospero forgiveness for having taken revenge, having concluded that reason and forgiveness are worth far more to his well-being than vengeance. Expressing one's final needs is the fourth step of nonviolent communication.

The words that invite one to open windows and not to build walls are found in the last lines of Prospero's dialogue, which speak of generosity and of an initial project that was 'to give pleasure.' Even though these words may not have worked out completely, Prospero asks us not only for emotional empathy, an understanding of the felt emotions, but also an epistemological empathy, which is a deeper kind of understanding that calls the audience to judge Prospero by his intentions, not solely based on his deeds. The audience is called, therefore, to become inhabitants of the island, alongside Prospero.

He takes one step back from his daughter, eventually leaving her the possibility to decide for her future life. Before, he was patronizing her, as her father and nobleman, and only at the end, he finally allows her to walk along her own path, freely pursuing love with its risks. He declares himself old and tired, understanding that the only way to leave the stormy place he lives is when the audience is deeply 'convinced' by his reasons. He assumes that the audience must perceive him, not only as a duke, as a father and a magician but as an ungrateful despot. By breaking the magic wand, symbolically he lets go of control, assuming a humble position towards the characters and the audience. Nonviolent communication does not leave room for pride and superiority but breaks them down.

1.5 Epilogue: Prosperous Unveiled

Shakespeare courageously brings in "The Tempest" the concepts of evil and good: 'Hell is empty, the devils are all here.' We must find the magical arts inside us, with us, if we need them to make peace with them, with ourselves, embracing forgiveness as the first solution.

By analogy, with many "devils" of our contemporary society, there is a greater need to sue style from NVC, choosing the right words; for example, not to say, "you are a total failure," but rather "I have noticed that your last activities could have been improved" or instead of saying in clinical practice, "this patient is better than you," replace this sentence with, "both of you are profoundly different." In everyday life, instead of saying "you are not listening to me," even if it is a true statement, we might suggest to rephrase it to "I am observing that you are using your mobile phone right now while I am talking," and lastly, instead of "get better soon," to a patient use, "here I am, is there something that would ease your pain?"

Let's also consider that nonviolent communication may not be possible for some "devils", but that does not mean hell has to be reopened; just stay away from it. Or at least acknowledge and be aware that there could be a narcissistic megalomaniac person in front of you, even though they will never listen and will compete with you in a violent communication style. Narcissists usually give orders, devalue deeds, and use sarcasm to bully others, not appreciating emotions, but instead gaslighting their main target in front of others. They make you feel wrong, inadequate, and worthless. If we wish, we can give them a chance or two chances for trying to have a fruitful conversation, but please be aware that we might foresee a glimpse of light, but this spark rarely lasts. In most cases, we only see darkness when communicating with narcissists. At least we have tried, and we should not take it personally. Prospero was wounded, took revenge for some time, but was never a narcissist and this is proved by the fact that ultimately, he asked our forgiveness; a narcissist will never get on his knees, remaining in a violent posture.

In our age which suffers from the imperative slogan "everything has to be politically correct", we run the risk to rush into superficial relationship with everyone and anyone: the word *connection* is polysemic. On the one hand, healthcare professionals aim is to establish "a real connection" between each other and with patients and caregivers, that is based on trust and intimacy, but, on the other hand, in the vernacular, mainly business world, this term is referred to knowing people, for example, in LinkedIn, they are generally mere contacts and not real listeners and helpers. And again, this holds true in the number of friends on Facebook: how many of our hundreds of contacts are real friends? This is a total misuse of the word friendship. Both kinds of "connections" are useful, one related to being in a professional, "pseudo-friendship" net, and the other is an human competence, the ability to create intimacy, affiliation, and intersubjectivity.

Sometimes, one needs the magic wand of Prospero to make the twist, to find the keys to enter the others' hearts: some of the people display a different pattern of the brain that explain why people are more violent in communication and why others are keener to the listening [10]. There are techniques form NVC and Narrative medicine which can be learned to develop trust and empathy, especially in difficult situations.

"The Tempest" is the legacy that Shakespeare leaves us, his last work before dying. It reminds us that our passage is ephemeral: "We are made of the same stuff as dreams, and of our wishes, and in the space and time of a dream is gathered our brief life," in the finale of Act IV.

7Let us not linger in resentment, but let's look at the facts, ask for justice, express our needs, speak out our needs with kindness and lightness, as Ariel teaches Prospero.

Now we can see that Bia, that violence in ancient Greek, goes in backstage, and Nike, the winged Victory goddess, light as Ariel, enters the scene, singing her song for having quit violence, and promoted peace conversations and peaceful deeds.

1.6 Practice Time

1. What is violence for you? And could you use a metaphor to explain it?
2. If you wish, read the epilogue of the "Tempest": highlight the "violent words" and the "nonviolent words."
3. Would you like to invent a different ending for the "Tempest"?
4. Think of your career as a student, resident, doctor, or health care worker, what was one of the most violent communications you had in your professional life?

    (a) Write some lines without caring about the wrongs or rights, just to capture the experience. Which emotions do you feel after having written in a venting way?
    (b) Now think that experience bearing in mind the four steps of NVC: Observation (fact checking), Emotions (Of the others and of the self), Needs (of the others and of the self), Request (words used to express the personal needs on both sides)
    (c) Do you envision any possibility of changing the outcome of this conversation, or do you think that any strategy could have been impossible?
    (d) If, from the other side, there were "walls" in communication, how do you feel now after having processed what happened with this method?

5. Would you like to read or re-read The Tempest after these dedicated lines?
6. Please review the following table (Table 1.1) that lists the natural primes of the Natural Sematic Language (NSM), try to use these supposed universal terms, as we have been using them to understand the word "violence" and the pronoun "we" [11].

Table 1.1 The Natural Semantic Metalanguage primes

Category	Primes
Substantives	I, you, someone, people, something/thing, body
Relational substantives	Kind, part
Determiners	This, the same, other~else~another
Quantifiers	One, two, some, all, much/many, little/few
Evaluators	Good, bad
Descriptors	Big, small
Mental predicates	Think, know, want, don't want, feel, see, hear
Speech	Say, words, true
Actions, events, movement	Do, happen, move
Existence, possession	Be (somewhere), there is, be (someone/something), (is) mine
Life and death	Live, Die
Time	When/time, now, before, after, a long time, a short time, for some time, moment
Space	Where/place, here, above, below, far, near, side, inside, touch (contact)
Logical concepts	Not, maybe, can, because if
Intensifier, augmentor	Very, more
Similarity	Like, as, way

References

1. Shakespeare, William. The tempest. In: Gill R, editor. 4th ed. London: Oxford University Press; 2001.
2. Rosenberg MB. Nonviolent communication: a language of life. 3rd ed. Puddle Dancer Press; 1998.
3. Varsou O. Teaching, research, innovation and public engagement. Chem: Springer; 2023.
4. WHO. n.d.. https://www.who.int/groups/violence-prevention-alliance/approach.
5. Marini, Maria Giulia, The languages of care in narrative medicine; 2019.
6. Trief PM, Uschner D, Kalichman S, Anderson BJ, Fette LM, Wen H, Bulger JD, Weinstock RS. Psychosocial factors predict medication adherence in young adults with youth-onset type 2 diabetes: longitudinal results from the TODAY2 iCount study. Diab Med. 2023;40(5):e15062.
7. Marini MG, Volpato E, Reale L, Portaro M, Uglietti A. Narratives on vaccination at the time of Covid-19. J Clin Studies. 2022;
8. Protests over Italy's Covid 'Green Pass' draw only scattered crowds. The New York Times (nytimes.com)
9. John, Donne. Meditation XVII. Devotions upon emergent occasions, and severall steps in my sicknes; n.d.
10. Iain MGC. The master and his emissary: the divided Brain and the making of the Western World. Yale University Press; 2019.
11. Goddard C, Wierzbicka A, editors. Meaning and universal grammar: theory and empirical findings. Amsterdam: John Benjamins; 2002.

Chapter 2
How Many Narrative Medicines Are in the History of Human Beings?

2.1 Language, the History of Its Use

In his book *Sapiens: A brief history of Humankind* [1], Yuval Noah Harari states and points out when in our Sapiens human species, cousin of chimpanzees, the Cognitive Revolution occurred so that the Sapiens could become stronger than tigers, giant animals and Neanderthal humankind: around 70,000 years ago. The Cognitive Revolution would have been followed by the Agricultural Revolution 10,000 years ago, the Scientific Revolution 500 years ago, and the Industrial Revolution 200 years ago.

Before exploring how the Cognitive Revolution occurred, let me tell the reader that *Sapiens* is a masterpiece if someone wants to learn empathy and collaboration, crossing through the 466 pages of the history of our species, with the facts, our fallacy in decision making, our genial ideas, our beliefs, and the subtle balance or unbalancing between the individual, the society, and the environment.

Seventy thousand years ago, the Cognitive Revolution started. Guess what it was based on? Language. Quite an easy answer for scholars, teachers, or fans of narrative and storytelling. Neuroscientists and archaeologists proved that language shaped the identity of the Sapiens and of the world before Harari wrote this book. However, he adds a unique point of view, which is an eye-opener to understand why Sapiens won and Neanderthal lost supremacy, although we know that we are intertwined. Neanderthal, according to Harari, had factual language based on true events: *Today I saw a lion, and we have to be careful*. This was the Neanderthal language: deeds, objective facts, chronicles. The Sapiens, which at that time (70,000 years ago) were still hunter-collectors as the Neanderthals, could have this kind of language: *Today I saw a lion: it said to me that if we are going to hunt for him, the whole spirit of the savannah will seek for revenge: however, if we sacrifice him, and kill him giving a tribute to the savannah and its gods, we might be praised*. On top of the real event "the seen lion," the Sapiens had and demonstrate imaginative

© The Author(s), under exclusive license to Springer Nature Switzerland AG 2024
M. G. Marini, *Non-violent Communication and Narrative Medicine for Promoting Sustainable Health*, New Paradigms in Healthcare,
https://doi.org/10.1007/978-3-031-58691-0_2

power, notice how she/he created a story, a myth, with a meta-objective that goes far beyond simply killing the lion. This story implies a possible war with the savannah and its gods. *We might be praised*, the Sapiens added this fantastic concept, but also of the possibility, the "may be." And, in fact, Sapiens left Africa since the tiers were too dangerous and went to other lands…But this is another story.

Flexibility and imagination are the two engines that brought Sapiens to subdue the Neanderthal and to end up until now. According to Harari's theory of Cognitive Revolution, stories and myths that related to actual facts were the fuel of the hunter-collectors to control bigger societies and are still here as a sociological need. Harari goes on across millenniums and centuries and brings us to our contemporaneity with a critical evaluation of what the Sapiens did but with one strong argument, affirming that the tipping point was the Cognitive Revolution, **the skill of narrating and creating stories**.

> In 2022, a wonderful Nobel Prize in Medicine was awarded to Svante Paabo [2] for founding paleo-genomics, the science that studies' the genes of our ancestors, and he has succeeded in uncovering the enchantment of the interweaving of early humans. Ancient DNA has confirmed that we are embedded in a rich history of human diversity and still embody it. In addition to the Sapiens genetic material, we have acquired 'laterally' other genes through interbreeding with Neanderthals and other species: a recent study has found that less than 10% of our genome is distinctive of Neanderthal, who evolved uniquely in us.
>
> The realization that the very essence of the Neanderthals, alongside the known Sapiens, is still present today—in every human heart, be it beating with fear or joy—has created a new emotional bond not only with them but also with all our other ancestors. We are truly an evolved and resilient weave beyond all wars, plagues, famines, and possible diseases.
>
> The Neanderthal DNA present in our DNA today proves that human beings have been able to create belonging, including different populations. As an analogy, the Romans included and did not erase the Etruscan population, embracing many of their beliefs and rituals, from divination to the building of arches to the deities on the Latin Pantheons.
>
> Nevertheless, history is told by the winners, as in this case, the Sapiens won with the skills of imagination and the skill to control wider groups of people through storytelling. Professor Robin Dunbar [3], using the average human brain size and considering the results of primates, proposed that humans can comfortably maintain 150 stable relationships. He theorized that this limit is a direct function of relative neocortex size and that this, in turn, limits group size. This threshold imposed by neocortical processing capacity is simply on the number of individuals with whom a stable interpersonal relationship can be maintained. On the periphery, the number also includes past colleagues,

> such as high school friends, with whom a person would want to reacquaint himself/herself if they met again. The control of higher group was achieved by storytelling, and, as Prof. Dunbar adds, the brewery had a tremendous impact: people gathered around the fire, and that alcohol—if moderate, could be an excellent endorphin-releasing factor, developing creativity and phantasy.

2.2 Between Factual and Symbolic Language in Healthcare

What have these to do with Medical Humanities and **Narrative Medicine**? Chronicles of facts are requested to take care of a patient. However, in the spoken and written narratives, we collect "factions," a neologism created from real events, the "facts" woven together also with fictitious thoughts (maybe true for the person who has a creed in them), conversations, things, the "fictions." In sciences and medical studies, we have been told to rely only on real facts; I *saw a lion today*, and discard other stories, *The gods of the savannah*, since we do not believe in their existence. However, this is very often just a point of view, that of the "Neanderthals" specifically. According to Harari, if we want to be good carers, we must accept the "faction" stories, which might occur during the visit, in the clinical setting, during home visits, or wherever that patient decides to tell us the pathography, that is the story of his/her illness.

If Harari stresses out the point that myth was there for social control, personally I think that illness, ageing, birth, and death put us in a fragile and vulnerable situation and fosters existential questions. We seek comfort in imagination and fantasy with spirituality beliefs (from God(s), to quantum physics and energetic levels). It is an individual inner drive, not only a story that we absorb by the external "media of communication". An inner silence which brings us not only to the clue of awareness but also to fantastic realms of our individuality in interaction with the others. Patients, since they live their illness experience, despite the reductionist approach which calls the disease with a technical name (i.e., Alzheimer Disease, Guillaume Barré Syndrome, COVID-19 Infection, etc.), might encounter the courage to "fight the lion" with the allied gods: someone calls it storytelling, belief, mind attitude, or placebo, but this works in terms of patient's outcomes, as we will read.

Let us make clear that in patients, the disease is there and the body aches. So, if "the lion is there" in people's mind, we have to choose what to do: escaping, if we know how to escape, taming the lion, or killing it (and many other creative possibilities). The objective loss of health is there and brings pain to patients' body, but what make the person with less functionality experiencing the pathway of care is the language, which mirrors the mindset of how people address the disease [4].

The reductionist providers of care often could not see and refuse to face the individual need for the *factions*. They claim relying on physical evidence to be the only legitimate fountain of knowledge, then go as far as labeling patients as ignorant liars and confused people. They believe that science brings the only truth that matters, and patient's voice can be a disturbing bias from the scientific true. What about if the carers could instead finetune with the patient's factions to understand the symbolic language used in conjunction with the facts?

We could distinguish two levels of fictions: the first one, related to the mirroring of the language used by the patient probably, looks more ethical according to our western dogma of clinical intervention. Let us "create" a possible dialogue between a patient and a doctor using the "faction" genre:

"This disease is a lion", the patient states,
"Yes, we have a lion in your body," the doctor replies.
"What can we do?" the patient asks.
"Making it dormant, and taming, we cannot definitely kill it, because there is no adequate weapon, since your body is the land where the lion lives, and also the land will be devastated by the blasters," the doctor explains, keeping on using this metaphoric language.
"Taming process, with what? With whom? How long it will take?" The patient asks.
"With me by your side, together with the team, with particular therapeutic options, with the things you cherish the most, and it will be a long process, since you have to learn a new style of life, but always with me at your side; living with this tamed dormant big cat inside you, it will become not dangerous...we will not call anymore a lion." The doctor tracks the patient's fear of having a lion inside the body.

This could be a sort of alignment between the carer and the patient. The metaphor is the *fil rouge* where, in this linguistic equation, the name *disease* is replaced by "*lion*", which could be transformed at the end of the dialogue in *a safe enough dormant big cat*. There is no lie, just a short storytelling which embellishes, gives meaning, provides solutions to the events, and softens the harshness of the violence of the beast, somehow taming it while keeping the right distance.

To make possible such an encounter, it is important to master the language and the art of listening: the carer could add another language to her/his technical jargon, the symbolic, fictional one. It is demonstrated that when we listen to a foreign language, our brain is more focused on the details of the words of the speaker because we fear to lose the meaning of what is told, and it is a challenging conversation [5]. This is a good tip for being able to really listen, imaging (again, once more the validity of imagination of the Sapiens) that we are listening to somebody who does not speak our native language.

2.3 Can Communication Alone Be More Effective Than Treatment Alone?

Eventually, the second level of fiction is to remove the existing treatment options for the illness and to leave only the storytelling. One may say, this is not an ethical practice. Right, we have to fix the boundaries about when to use only words, or when giving effective drugs to cure the disease. However, in 2014, researchers in Canada [6] did an outcome research study about the role of communication in the treatment of patients with chronic back pain. Half the patients in the study received mild electrical stimulation from physical therapists, and half received sham stimulation (all the equipment is set up, but the electrical current is never activated). Sham treatment — placebo — worked reasonably well with a noted 25% reduction in their levels of pain. The patients who got the real stimulation did even better since their pain levels decreased by 46%.

However, there was a sub-study, even more interesting, in which each of these groups was further divided into two halves. One half experienced only limited conversation from the therapist (retaining the "disease" mindset). With the other half, the healthcare provider asked open-ended questions and listened attentively to the answers (biography and pathography). They expressed empathy about the patients' situation and offered words of encouragement (i.e., *we will tame the lion*). Patients who underwent placebo treatment but had therapists who actively communicated reported a 55% decrease in their pain. *Communication alone was more effective than treatment alone.* The patients who got both electrical stimulation and a good conversation were the clear winners, with a 77% reduction of pain.

In **an editorial on the New York Time**, Dr. Ofri writes [7];

> *Frequently my patients ask if a multivitamin will give them more energy. In the past, I would say no, because there are no significant scientific studies to demonstrate this, and because in the absence of a vitamin deficiency there's not much for a basic multivitamin pill to do. Now I take a different approach. I say something along the lines of "Many of my patients find that they have more energy when they take a multivitamin." I'm not lying, because many have indeed said so. Without fail, there are always a few patients who come back at the next visit and swear they feel much better. Some argue that it is unethical to promote placebos to patients. But increasingly, many say it would be unethical not to give placebos a try in situations where patients are not getting relief from traditional means (and where it would not cause harm or replace a necessary treatment).*

Storytelling works for Sapiens. Sometimes it is not enough alone to counteract a severe condition with active drugs, for instance, in very subjective conditions such as pain the use of storytelling produces positive health outcomes. Factions work if integrated also with other good therapeutic options. As Ofri wrote, there are "Factions" of doctors (note the polysemic word, faction—the belonging to a group or faction, and a neologism formed by the connection and abbreviation of fact and fictions), those who are *pro placebo* stories, those who are *against placebo* stories. Again, it depends on the severity of the patient's condition, her/his background, their creeds, beliefs, and mindset, and not just for the one seeking a cure, but for doctors and carers since we are all, Sapiens behind the roles, even now, after 70,000 years.

And for the lovers of fiction, I wish to quote the words of Tyrion Lannister in the closure of Game of Thrones—I don't know if the screenwriters read Harari's History of Sapiens, nonetheless we all seem to hold to the same belief:

> *What unites people? Tyrion asked. Armies? Gold? Flags? No. It's stories, he said. There's nothing in the world more powerful than a good story. Nothing can stop it. No enemy can defeat it.*

As Jean-Do, affected by the locked-in syndrome, a quadriplegia that causes the inability to speak, so that the patient communicates with other through coded messages by blinking the eyes, in his cult illness memoir, *The Diving Bell and the Butterfly* [8], dictated only through the blinking process, a kind of Augmented Alternative Communication, notes: *"I will stop to complain: two things are still there, memory and imagination"*.

And with this imagination, he starts his interior dialogue that softens the hardship of his condition: storytelling, in this case, becomes his strategy for personal coping and not for political social control, creating propaganda. Story telling as Jerome Bruner writes in *Acts of Meaning* [9] is an immense powerful tool that we learn to mitigate our vulnerability, fragility, and difficult situation, since the world outside can be a *"hard world, and it's hard to get by, just upon a smile"* [10].

2.3.1 How Many "Narrative Medicines"? Helping Ourselves with the Name of the Rose

Narrative medicine is based on language, both of chronicles and storytelling, both verbal and nonverbal, both rational and emotional, looking backwards, to the here and now and forward. Are there institutional definitions for Narrative Medicine in the world? The most widely published is that one written by Professor Rita Charon, in USA at Columbia University, who created the "labelling" *Narrative Medicine*. This is Rita Charon definition: "medicine practiced with these skills of recognizing, absorbing, interpreting, and being moved by the stories of illness" (). Interestingly, parallel and quite synchronically to the creation of the term "Narrative Medicine" a similar definition arose in the UK, *Narrative-Based Medicine*, *"What happens between the doctor and the patient"* in the end of the last century and the beginning of the new millennium. In Italy, we have the guidelines issued by the Institute *Superiore di Sanità* which defines Narrative Medicine as "a communication skill to improve the diagnostic and therapeutic care pathway".

During the last years, a fruitful but sometimes burdensome dialogue was there to set this gemstone in a single frame and become the sole owner of this discovery.

Personally, using the analogy with the book 'The Name of the Rose' written by Umberto Eco [11], writer and semiologist, I tried, to explain that -whether we call these topics' Humanities for Health' or 'Medical Humanities' or 'Narrative Medicine', or 'Narrative-Based Medicine', or 'Narrative-Based Practice'—we all share the joint mission of serving the health and wellbeing of the person living an illness or vulnerability condition, the healthcare professional, the caregivers, the decision makers and the citizenship too.

The Name of the Rose novel is built on three layers of reading. The most evident is that of an entertaining novel about a series of murders in an abbey, with a detective, the Franciscan friar William of Baskerville; the second layer is the historical one, with an accurate description of life in an abbey during the Middle Ages, introducing the readers to the minds of monks and peasants of that time. The third level (and here the semiologist Umberto Eco comes out), is a philosophical one, related to the philosophy of language. The thriller ends with this sentence, *'Stat rosa pristinae nomine, nomina nuda tenemus.*' Which translates to "Originally, there was a rose, but we have only its naked name." We can hardly grasp what a rose is, by its name alone, and this applies to the names of events, facts, objects, feelings, thoughts, and beliefs. If we can only superficially understand *one* rose, how could we define in a unique way, more than 30,000 thousand subspecies of roses living on this planet? Could this be true of the many forms and applications of Narrative Medicine, and to the Health Humanities, which probably had their birth in a mythological age, since there are so many myths about health and illness, and gods and goddesses related to this unique existential matter. There is no possibility of holding tight onto only one name, because names are just pale description of life.

In *The Name of the Rose*, there are two main thinking trends: those of the innovators and those of the status quo. Umberto Eco puts the readers in the middle of a dispute between William of Baskerville—innovative and humble, the person who says in the end '…nomina nuda tenemus'—and Bernardo Gui, a Dominican friar inquisitor, emissary of the established church, a global controller, against any change. Gui is sure that all the necessary names are there, and that no new names should be created, since this would have been heretical, given the right number of words by God. Even more, their use should occur only controlled in a top-down way, by the center of power at that time (the establishment of the Church). In the novel, there is a continuous dynamic between dogma, bigotry and moralism on the one hand and ethics, discovery and compassion fact-checking the other side.

There is a hidden character, the blind friar Jorge, who is the "guardian of 'knowledge'" (he is the master of the library maze), and he is a symbol for not seeing what is happening around him in terms of figurative signs and needed language. He, together with Bernardo Gui, is also the owner of an old dogmatic culture, which argues against the production of future books and promotes solely the reproduction of old texts.

Now if we refer to the *EBM-cracy,* we can understand how futile is to argue for labelling Narrative Medicine or Health Humanities, or Medical Humanities of Narrative-Based Medicine in this age of technocracy that strips subjects of their meaning, creating an increasingly narrower space of being.

It is a violent act to be banished as a "heretic" because we can choose one approach to Narrative Medicine, or worse than this, being undervalued by the world of EBM (Evidence-based Medicine), which sometimes considers Health Humanities a waste of time. I write these lines, because I am quite confident that you, the reader, someday will have to face the fact that someone will bring the blind faith in Science to an end. I would like to raise awareness of this risk, as many of us scholars of the humanities are aware of the arrogant and violent styles of communication that exist inside and outside the practice of medicine. William of Baskerville is a Master of Nonviolent communication: fact checking, understanding emotions the other might have felt and the needs behind the emotions, and the verbalizations of the requests, despite the limits of freedom given by the church at that time.

Eco suggests, in the end with the discovery of lightness, the simple act of a smile possesses great power. A good send of humor, which Aristoteles praised in his book on Comedy, combined with art can provide a new ground for finding synergies across cultures. The Greek philosopher has a plural voice, writing both on Tragedy and on Comedy, melting together diverse emotions.

Analogically, Health Humanities and Narrative Medicine are worthy of evolution, with different names, according to the contexts, and remembering that every patient or person is a world apart. This universal concept has to be put in the original cultural context: we have diverse languages, peoples, beliefs, values, interests, religions, economies, welfare systems, ways to provide health, caring and curing, life and death. Only a plurality of approaches which encompass the different ways of thinking about Narrative Medicine and Humanities for Health and its integration with EBM can be the key for a harmonized approach.

I have sometimes been imprisoned by this violent dispute on what this "rose" is; we call it maybe Narrative Medicine, Humanities for Health or Narrative-Based Medicine. There are indeed different cultures and schools, here in Europe and in America, Australia, and elsewhere. So many roses forming a wonderful rose garden, and all we can do is stand in awe, overwhelmed by the beauty of these scents, the variety of colors, the shapes of the petals. Moreover, I recalled my reading *The Name of the Rose*, and I concluded that if we can allow ourselves to smile and laugh, although disputes do happen because they are part of professional life, with lightness, we can try to release the burden of some words, and even erase the word "heretic" from the conversation. which is nowadays untold in public but is unfortunately acted violently during gossip and on social media, as that one of today, read fresh on Facebook: "this could displease many others, but I was told to be the Italian excellence of Narrative Medicine in the field of Palliative Care": written exactly with this words, with no publication—for me fact-checking—behind, just an authoritative self-affirmation, that made me smile.

Smile, laugh and not use the slowing down pace and the art of watching the polyphonic signs taught by William of Baskerville to his novice Adso from Melk.

Narrative medicine plurality of visions should somehow compact together, since in congresses, academies, the media, hospitals, and in every care setting, if healthcare providers reveal that they are use a narrative-based approach in their practice, they may be perceived as not "evidence-based enough", therefore, lacking scientific competence.

If healthcare providers do follow an evidence-based approach, they have an easier life in this *EBM-cratic* world, but they will lack an incredible tool developed over these thousand years: the power of combining the factual and symbolic language, our most ancient and rich vocabulary, capable of building individual stories to mitigate the violence of illness, *when the lions come*.

2.4 Practice Time

1. Would you like to give your definition of the word "story"?
2. Would you like to give your definition of "chronicle"?
3. Would you like to say what Health Humanities are for you?

4. Would you like to say what Medical Humanities are for you?
5. Would you like to say what is Narrative Medicine for you?
6. "Stat rosa, pristina nomine, nomina nuda tenemus"; the original rose remains only in its name; we hold only bare names. Would you like to run a short reflective writing on this statement, on the impossibility of capturing the meaning of names with current language?
7. Have you encountered a situation in which you have felt stigmatized, or labeled a "heretic" for believing in the power of Health Humanities and Narrative Medicine? How did you act or react?

References

1. Harari YN. Sapiens: a brief history of human kind. Sapiens: A Brief History of Humankind; 2011.
2. Callaway E. From Neanderthal genome to Nobel prize: meet geneticist Svante Pääbo. Nature. 2022;
3. Dunbar R. How many friends does one person need? Dunbar's number and other evolutionary quirks. Faber & Faber; 2011.
4. Marini MG. The languages of care in narrative medicine. Springer; 2019.
5. Pérez A, Dumas G, Karadag M, Duñabeitia JA. Differential brain-to-brain entrainment while speaking and listening in native and foreign languages. Cortex. 2018;
6. Fuentes J, Armijo-Olivo S, Funabashi M, Miciak M, Dick B, Warren S, Rashiq S, Magee DJ, Gross DP. Enhanced therapeutic alliance modulates pain intensity and muscle pain sensitivity in patients with chronic low back pain: an experimental controlled study. Phys Ther. 2014:477–89.
7. Danielle Ofri. The conversation placebo. The New York Times; 2017
8. Bauby, Jean Dominique. The diving bell and the butterfly, paperback, 1998
9. Bruner J. Acts of meaning. Harvard University Press; 1993.
10. Charon R. Narrative medicine: honoring the stories of illness. Oxford University Press; 2006.
11. Eco, Umberto. The name of the rose; 1980.

Chapter 3
Communicating Science to Citizens, Patients, and Doctors: The Violence of Becoming Dogmatic

This chapter is a tribute to Piero Angela, who in Italy opened the door to scientific divulgation through the media. His wish was to introduce the Italian population to biology, medicine, and Science in general. Piero Angela was born in Turin on December 22, 1928, and died in Rome on August 13, 2022. He was the most distinguished Italian popularizer of science, television host, and essayist.

From the beginning of the 1970s, Angela also devoted himself to creating television programs dedicated to science divulgation, with his first being "Destination Man," in 1971, aimed at a broad audience. The series "Quark" started in 1981, which was noted for its curious title that came from a term used in physics, which was coined by scientists studying hypothetical subnuclear particles to define what were considered the smallest possible building blocks of matter. The metaphor of Quark so was to investigate biology through little, tiny but core elements, and, as well to travel inside nature [1].

"Quark's" formula was particularly innovative at the time because all the available technological means and the resources of television communication were deployed to make the complex topics discussed familiar. For example, documentaries by the BBC and David Attenborough, cartoons by Bruno Bozzetto used to explain the most difficult concepts, interviews with experts set out in the most precise and daily life-based language compatible with the complexity of the topics, and explanations in the studio.

He began his career as a radio reporter, later becoming an envoy and establishing himself as the anchorman of the RAI news program; however, he remains best known as the creator and presenter of Anglo-Saxon-style popularization programs, with which he gave life to a new documentary strand of Italian television and a unique style of scientific journalism, expressed in numerous non-fiction publications. Official honors were paid to him for the important work of bringing the public closer to the world of culture and science carried out over much of his life. His last words left a legacy to all Italian citizens- however, I think that they can be expatriated in many other countries:

> *Dear friends, I am sorry I am no longer with you after 70 years together. But nature also has its rhythms. These have been very stimulating years for me, which have led me to get to know the world and human nature.*
>
> *Above all, I was lucky enough to meet people who helped me realize what every person would like to discover. Thanks to Science and a method that allows one to approach problems rationally and humanely.*
>
> *Despite a long illness, I managed to complete all my programs and projects (even a small satisfaction: a jazz record on the piano). But also, sixteen episodes dedicated to the school on environmental and energy issues.*
>
> *It was an extraordinary adventure, lived intensely and made possible thanks to the collaboration of a great group of authors, collaborators, technicians, and scientists.*
>
> *In my turn, I have tried to give back what I learned.*
>
> *Dear all, I have done my part. Try to do yours too for this difficult country of ours.*
>
> *A big hug*
>
> *Piero Angela* [2].

A common Italian experience is growing up watching "Quark" on Saturday evenings with family, and many of us were so enchanted by the beauty of science with its unknowns that we have likely chosen a scientific career also because of his tremendous work. Piero Angela fought superstition but was always willing to understand the roots of some superstitions. He was a strong believer in rationality, but before the unknown things, he never fell in an over-rationalization process. He admitted that science had so much more to discover, and that it "never" gives certainties but probabilities, sometimes better odds and sometimes worse odds.

He commented on COVID-19 negationists and those who brushed aside the seriousness of the SARS-related disease, taking a position out of the blaming culture of many scientists against NO-.Vax population, trying to find the reasons for these open negations: *"Maybe they have been treated as "donkeys"*. To whom does Angela refer to? The scientific experts, their doctors, the institutions. Piero Angela would never have treated any person as inept in learning and understanding, including the population of people who rejected or were hesitant before the vaccination.

"Better trying to persuade them, persisting with patience, of the existence of the virus, giving them scientific data", Piero Angela stated. The blaming culture used on hesitancy on vaccination was useless and a booster of violence, as shown by the riots in the streets of many Italian and European cities.

He had a wise, balanced strategy of communication; unfortunately, many did not exemplify the same eloquence and poise in media communication during the convulsive 2020, 2021, and 2022 period.

3.1 "Science Says So"

"Science says so" is an apodictic statement, leaving no room for any interlocution, which is all too often used on today's talk shows, in newspaper reports, and as clickbait in video thumbnails.

3.1 "Science Says So"

Behind this verbalization, the assumption is that something is true just because "science says so." This reasoning comes from several doctors who are also responsible for our health policies, and it is expressed as if we were called to an act of Faith since a truth demonstrated by science becomes indissoluble, irrefutable, and surrounded by an aura of eternity. I do not wish to go into the issues that have recently divided the country, where this meaning of "science" has been sharpened against the most boorish denialism, but with respect to the scientific method of the 19th century, which rests precisely on the questioning of the statement *"Sicut scientia locutus est,"* "thus science spoke," taking up the Latin language, speaking of Science in an ecclesiastical way. If Science says so, let us be careful; it is a certain truth.

In the philosophy of science of the last few centuries, we do not enter an abstract world of words divorced from the method, but on the contrary, we put ourselves into the method: positivism is based on the Galilean method, once a hypothesis has been formulated and verified, the scientific thesis is valid.

In the 18th century, the philosopher David Hume came in to refute this very wave of positivism by introducing the concept of probability. Do you remember Hume? He is the philosopher who brings disquiet, and as Immanuel Kant would later say of him, he is the one who "woke him up from his dogmatic sleep". David Hume offers only good probabilities that the sun might rise tomorrow on earth, but no certainty. In fact, even if we do not want to think about it too much, who knows what could happen within our microcosm of the solar system? In the film that is so controversial, *"Don't Look Up"*, the sun will continue to rise, but we humans will no longer even question it. However, Hume also shows us an exit to this dismal existential question providing a counterargument: It is reasonable to doubt, but doubting unconditionally would no longer get us out of bed in the morning, with or without the sun around the earth.

In the 1930s, the Science of certainty and determinism was shaken up when Heisenberg, with his Principle of Indeterminacy, stated that there could be no objectivity but that at the very moment we are experimenting, we become part of the participatory universe and thus fatally change the fate of the experiment. We interfere. We cannot be a pure observer.

This is not a trivial matter because we are also called into play with our subjectivity of choice of what we want to study and observe, and therefore, by opening other doors to these lines, what research do we want to finance. New vaccines? New genetic precision medicine to understand why there are people who do not get infected with COVID-19, despite being in constant contact with those who test positive for the disease? Vaccines are considered fundamental and effective; in the second phase of the pandemic they were hailed as the only possible way out. But are they? And will they be sufficient on their own, since the alpha and delta variants of the Coronavirus have been replaced by totally different viruses, the Omicron Beta 5 and many other different ones? Those vaccines were developed for a deadly and aggressive pulmonary disease of the alpha and beta variants, and they are of moderate utility facing this superspreading virus, which is thankfully much less lethal at a pulmonary level than other diseases of the same class. Who decides where to allot the money for research? This too, is pure human subjectivity, the direction that scientific research takes is often determined by collective interests. as well as collective interests. In a global welfare system where citizens contribute through the tax system, there should be a transparent method to choose, maybe based on deliberative democracy (https://academic.oup.com/edited-volume/28086 [3]. Meanwhile, COVID-19 research funding dominated the world, MIT in Boston has published research that [4] shows how hearing loss not only can benefit of hearing aids but can be reversed to a certain extent, acting with an advanced technology, and this discovery drew my attention.

About 8,5% of the population aged between [5] 56 and 65, so perfectly fitting in a productivity age, experience hearing loss. Isn't this a high prevalence condition that brings to disability? This reflection is not just a complaint per se, but we must bring clarity to where funding for research is being invested.

Let us return to the "scientific method" in the strict sense of the term: Karl Popper, 'the great scientific preacher' of the last century, insisted that something can be true from a scientific point of view until it is falsified according to his theory, one would say "until proven otherwise". Analogue within *dubio pro reo*, from Roman Law: better a guilty man out in the society than an innocent man in jail. With this analogy, Karl Popper, the father of knowledge falsification theory, tells us that it is better to think we are guilty and, therefore, to accept and identify our cognitive bias as scientists so as not to generate false knowledge a priori, theories that we just love (and it is so human to fall in love with our own theories and wish for them to be true). However, they are partial, and knowledge proceeds by falsification. So, it is standard practice in research to assume that what we are looking for is not true, formation of a null hypothesis, to interfere as little as possible with the experiment.

For Popper, in fact, there is a rigorous and precise method aimed at containing the cognitive distortions, among which are self-affirmation bias, or the desire to be right. Self-affirmation bias can manifest in research as a desire for an experiment to end as we expect it to. It is a method based on the null hypothesis, for instance a null hypothesis could be that "there is no difference between the two therapeutic paths under scrutiny." With probabilities and never with certainties. Karl Popper would never have said, "Science says so," but he would have said, with probability, that this drug works in a certain percentage of the population, until proven otherwise or until new discoveries are made.

The Austrian philosopher Paul Feyerabend, a pupil of Popper, wrote an essay with Imre Lakatos, 'For and against the method'. Unfortunately, Lakatos passed away prematurely, but the two opened an open Socratic dialogue, supporting the "pros" (Lakatos) and "cons" (Feyerabend) of the scientific method, to arrive eventually in bounding a marvelous final synergy, where methodological rigidity and anarchy—as Feyerabend calls it—of being a scientist coexist.

If there had not been freedom and anarchy, we would still be believing in ancient dogmas based in geocentrism; we would not have discovered the therapy of relativity, and the world would be the one described by Dante in the sky of fixed stars. It is precisely during the Copernican Revolution that Feyerabend affirms that the dogma collapsed [6]. The violent forms of resistance that were used to defend the geocentric dogma was there, torturing and imprisoning scientists, burning them on rogues as heretics (again) together with strong women-defined witches.

The cultural and scientific paradigm changes at a slow pace. Innovators do exist, and they are those who try alternative routes never previously taken or make associations through the observation of phenomena they see with new eyes, through the principle of serendipity, accidental discoveries, which are nothing more than an extraordinary associative creativity process. Take for example, Fleming's famous discovery of Penicillin, or equally famous, the chance discovery of the Americas, convinced that he had circumnavigated the earth and arrived in the Indies.

We cannot anticipate the future, but we can cite examples from the past. Consider how treatment for gastric ulcers in the 1970s was restricted to gastro-resection surgery because there were no drugs. Gradually, pharmacologists developed antihistamines (H2 antagonists), then proton pump inhibitors, and finally, around the end of the 20th century, Barry Marshall and Robin Warren discovered that Helicobacter pylori, a bacterium, is the cause of the gastric ulcer. For this discovery, they received the Nobel Prize, much later, in 2005. Therapies have followed, first the antibiotic, and now the intake of probiotics to eradicate Helicobacter pylori. A new therapeutic paradigm is here that was unthinkable in the days when surgeons had to intervene.

Another example is neuroplasticity, which was once thought by neuroscientists to manifest only during childhood [7] but research in the latter half of the 20th century showed that many aspects of the brain can be altered (or are "plastic") even throughout adulthood. Stigma was very strong during the last century among neuroscientists who were studying the potential of neuroplasticity in adults, but we know that to prevent cognitive decline, high literacy and engagement in culturally demanding activities are beneficial. Why? Cognitive activities involve the continual creation of new brain connections, resulting in a so-called "cognitive reserve" capable of counteracting the effects of damage to certain brain circuits. This has led to an increase in promotion of engagement in mind-stimulating activities (learning new languages, playing a musical instrument, reading books, or even more simply being engaged in a stimulating job or pastime, as well as participating in social and recreational activities) as a possible strategy for delaying the onset of Dementia in individuals with initial cognitive decline. The findings on adult neuroplasticity in the past century was barely mentioned among the establishment scientists while the innovators continued to search for this possibility, and new technologies brought the evidence that the innovators needed.

The reality is very complex, and I would like to stress that these discoveries have a certain likelihood, in other words, they do not guarantee true things but probable events today. Feyerabend argues that our brain should not be bridled only in the methodological rituals of research because the conditioning is too rigid, but instead, it is in the maximum chaos where we have all degrees of freedom to create and innovate. In his essay, Feyerabend goes on to verify the role that Science has taken on in Western society: Science, to a certain extent, has become a repressive ideology, even though it began as a liberation movement, and the philosopher thought that society should protect itself from an excessive influence of science, just as it protects itself from other ideologies.

Starting from the assumption that there is no universal, ahistorical scientific method, Feyerabend deduced that Science does not deserve its *"overrated privileged role"* in Western society since scientific views do not arise from the use of a universal method that guarantees consistently high-quality conclusions, or ethicality. In fact, he was one of the first to denounce that Science had become an ideology, a faith.

The method, the yardstick, serves and is a fundamental tool, and we cannot give permission to the deniers to invalidate its usefulness; we know, and I want to emphasize that the vaccines work, but alone are not enough. Recalling that there are, unfortunately, also many diseases for which there is neither a diagnosis nor a cure.

Churchill states, "It has been said that democracy is the worst form of government, except for all those forms that have been tried so far." This irony can be married with the Science of Popper and his method, knowing that it is extremely improbable, leaving room for creativity, disengaging from research only in the short-term and aimed at immediate profit (drugs or vaccines with 3–6 months of efficacy), because it is too steeped in protocols, and becoming freer from the screaming of the inquisitor of faith who in the TV talk show repeats as a litany the phrase, "Science says so." Maybe listening to the narratives of the people could help in building more trustful and informed relations of care, as Piero Angela was teaching us, "Don't treat people as donkeys."

3.2 The Blaming Culture and Hesitancy Towards Vaccination

In a democracy, everyone has the right to voice their concerns about an illness, a treatment, or a cure, although not fully knowledgeable on the specific subject, but just based on *opinion and personal experience*. Everyone has the possibility to declare their position and the reasons for accepting or rejecting a specific health-related topic that policymakers must listen to. Decision-makers can decide on specific routes to undertake, but they should also consider alternative positions. Therefore, the decision could be top-down, but the consultation act is bottom-up. We are entering into the edgy field of narrative bioethics, which implies the internal (and external) debate that occurs when one is posed with an important decision to make. Acts can only be called moral when they are post-conventional (chosen after the convention), inner-directed (defined on the autonomous values), and responsible (interdependent with the others) [8]. Such acts are autonomous in a new moral meaning. The goal of ethics (bioethics) is to promote post-conventional and mature human beings.

Even the WHO recognized that not every healthcare professional should automatically be considered full-fledged "believers" in the SARS-COV2 Vaccination program and wrote very meaningful guidelines on how to cope with Human Resources and Vaccines [9]:

As facilitators and channels to reach the public, health workers represented a resource and an opportunity to help achieve successful COVID-19 vaccination. However, fully leveraging health workers as positive influencers for COVID-19 vaccination was not straightforward. Health workers might have faced challenges related to vaccination of their patients, and some had concerns about vaccination themselves. Most health workers supported and promoted vaccination, but some faced structural, social, or personal barriers to doing so. This called for making continuous efforts to listen to health workers and understand the barriers and drivers they experience. *Passive forms of training such as written guidelines and education modules are less effective if they stand alone. Health Care practices are influenced by a dynamic interplay of social, professional, economic, political, and contextual factors in a changing environment.*

3.3 From the Violence of Social Pressure to the Finding of a Common "Good"

In 2021, Italian media and news networks, at a single level, and searching for easy polarizations, often took for granted the fact that the Vaccinated People were the "good ones" and the Hesitant or not vaccinated people the "bad ones". Without listening to the divergent stories (including hesitant doctors), we would have committed an immoral act according to narrative bioethics. Blaming and shaming cultures did not produce any change of positions towards vaccinations, but most likely contributed to the riots that were witnessed on the streets and burnout in healthcare professionals.

At ISTUD, we carried out 1 year of narrative-based research, "Narrating Covid-19 Vaccinations" [9] addressed to the public. The aim was to build a compass for orienting public health workers towards crafting vaccination campaigns consistent with the *why, the meanings, the values, and the narrative consistency*. Often, solutions "are all in the stories", as Martha Montello writes [10]. At the end of this research project, we found possible strategic solutions, respecting the individual, the public, and the healthcare providers. Instead of focusing, in an obsessive way, on the fight against the hesitant and those who completely refused the vaccination, the research a gave clear indication about what should have been communicated by the media. *Out of 356 narratives of vaccinated persons, the enthusiasts of the vaccination were only 35%.*

From the narratives, the metanarrative reasons for vaccination were *"not making my loved ones, my friends, others ill"*, besides the expected "getting back to having a social life", and secondarily but very distantly "not getting ill". In fact, vaccination was mainly perceived as a gesture of altruism, of building a common good. Based on these observations, the campaign could have been designed on a foundation of caring and tenderness towards others, avoiding directing blame towards who (which were only a few, so singling out this population, in my opinion, was a waste of time and money) were hesitant or rejected the procedure. I think that narrative medicine is a wonderful approach to exploring humans' attitudes and wishes.

3.4 Practice Time

1. With my students attending the Master in Applied Narrative Medicine program and the Master for Scientists, where I teach Communication borrowing from Linguistics, I have been using what I call the "Piero Angela's test." The students who just recently graduated with the dissertation of a thesis bearing a very "cryptic" name, "The Role of Substance Abracadabra on the Receptor PXYZ on murine cells to antagonize the effect of the cytokines XCCCCVVVVVVV," (I hope it's clear it's a phantasy name) are kindly asked to express the content of their work in easy terms. Everyone should understand, every citizen, from the housekeeper (with my full respect for the housekeeping, which is a hard job because you are always on board) to the Nobel Prize recipient. In the beginning, they launch themselves in the trial, and they fail. After the first three understandable words, they end up saying CRISPR, or hematocrit, or TLR2/4 receptor agonist in Chemotherapy.

    So, I ask them to reflect in silence, to think to layman's words, and if they must express a difficult name, always to let it be followed by a clear explanation or use of metaphors, and they succeed-- most of them saying, "I didn't know it was so difficult."

    Yes, good Communication requires art, discipline, good choice of words, and a confident posture while saying them. This is the test I love to practice with healthcare professionals (physicians, nurses, etc.) when they must explain a diagnosis and how a potential treatment works. Only through conveying in easily accessible language to the patient the diagnosis and the cure is it possible to create reciprocal trust which is the basis for shared decision making. Otherwise, patients may supinely consent and either a.) follow the rules without being aware of what they are doing, or b.) not adhere to treatment, possibly getting worse.

    In the age of the Internet Revolution, there are medically literate patients who show that they can speak and understand medical jargon. This is a very important first step, but if we want to cure not only the disease but also take care of the whole person according to the biological, psychological, social, and existential model, we could include daily symbolic language.

    Now it is up to you: think of one of the patients of your laboratory work as a researcher. Try to explain with easy words the name of the diagnosis, of the treatment, and of the research you are carrying out, if any. If thinking of a patient, try to figure out a dialogue between you and the patient based on a clear explanation, but also adding a warm tone. Whatever you would convey as news. Maybe this patient would ask from your scientific certainties: What would you say? What kind of certainties could you provide, if any?

2. Now think about Science- I know it is too vague, so think of a breathtaking scientific success. Why do you consider it a great success? Do you think that this success is forever? Has this success undermined previous scientific convictions? Try to apply reflective writing on this case, putting as the title the scientific success you have chosen.
3. In a democracy, you also have the power to decide how to invest money in research: in which field would you like to invest more? Could you narrate a justification, so that Venture capitalists could be interested in your idea?
4. What do you think about the practice of including citizens with diverse backgrounds (nationalities, socioeconomic history, education levels, etc.) in discussions surrounding the COVID-19 vaccination? Would you like to narrate your experience with your COVID-19 vaccination? Do you think that every citizen has the right to speak out? And if you had to persuade someone to receive the vaccination, what would you tell her/him?

References

1. https://it.wikipedia.org/wiki/Piero_Angela
2. https://www.rainews.it/articoli/2022/08/lultima-lettera-di-piero-angela-ho-fatto-la-mia-parte-fate-la-vostra-in-questo-difficile-paese-0c563a0a-be4a-4c71-88ff-58e2c83a9d2f.html
3. Bächtiger A, Dryzek JS, et al. The Oxford handbook of deliberative democracy. Oxford University Press; 2018.
4. https://www.nidcd.nih.gov/health/statistics/quick-statistics-hearing
5. Ho D. A philosopher goes to the doctor. Routledge; 2019.
6. Finocchiaro M. Science, method, and argument in Galileo: philosophical, historical and historiographical essays. Springer; 2021.
7. Diniz C, Crestani A. The times they are a-changin': a proposal on how brain flexibility goes beyond the obvious to include the concepts of "upward" and "downward" to neuroplasticity. Mol Psychiatry. 2023;
8. Gracia D. "Bioethics, from stories to history", medicine, healthcare and philosophy. Springer; 2005.
9. Health workers in focus: Policies and practices for successful public response to COVID-19 vaccination. WHO.
10. Monthello M. Narrative ethics, narrative ethics: the role of stories in bioethics, special report. Hastings Center Rep. 2014;44(1):S2–6.

Chapter 4
The Violence of the Loss and Lack of Rituals

Cherry-picking from literature, with analogue thinking, *we* will address the violence of the loss and lack of rituals using a Greek tragedy, Antigone. Who is Antigone? Daughter of Jocasta and Oedipus, thus of incest *par excellence*, Antigone is the protagonist of a tragedy written by Sophocles—*Antigone*, 422 BC.

Let us start analyzing her name: *Anti* means "against" and *Gono* "born," thus, literally a person "born against." Some scholars write, "born as a substitute," but this seems implausible given the life she led, which we shall soon see was a complete opposition to tyranny. Antigone has a sister, Ismene, and two brothers, Eteocles and Polynices, all incestuous children from Jocasta and Oedipus.

After accompanying her father, Oedipus, who blinded himself after he discovered the violation of this taboo, to his death at Colonus, Antigone decides to return to her city, Thebes. At this point, the war of the seven against the city had just begun, caused by discord between her brothers Eteocles and Polynices, who killed each other. Creon, the new king of Thebes, Jocasta's brother, issues a proclamation forbidding the burial of Polynices because he had allied himself for the battle against his brother with the city of Argos, leaving his body lying for the dogs.

Creon
…For Polyneices 'tis ordained that none
Shall give him burial or make mourn for him,
But leave his corpse unburied, to be meat
For dogs and carrion crows, a ghastly sight.
So am I purposed; never by my will
Shall miscreants take precedence of true men,
But all good patriots, alive or dead,
Shall be by me preferred and honored….

Antigone, disobeying Creon's orders, worthily buries her brother Polynices. To "bury" in this sense means to take the body, wash it, anoint it with oil, and then dig the grave to bury the corpse.

Antigone, the "Born Against" seeks help from her sister Ismene, and these are the words of Sophocles, writing the dialogue between them:

Antigone*: You can now show whether your soul is noble indeed or unworthy of your noble lineage.*
Ismene*: But if this is the case, my unhappy sister, what can I do or not do?*
Antigone*: You can share with me the burden of action...*
Ismene*: What action? What are you thinking of?*
Antigone*: ...and help me to lift the body....*
Ismene*: Do you want to bury him? Even if it is forbidden?*
Antigone*: He is my brother; he is also your brother. If you oppose, I will not betray him.*
Ismene*: But Creon forbids it, you wretch!*
Antigone*: He cannot separate me from the people I love.*

Her sister Ismene, whose name probably derives from a river flowing near Thebes, does not help her; on the contrary, she condemns and leaves her alone. Two different personalities, where possible, even a nonviolent communication approach would not have worked, but this is the genesis of the tragedy. Antigone is left alone to lift the corpse, bury it, and raise her voice against the tyrant Creon on the abomination of the law against the burial of enemies to his reign.

The "Born Against," lacking the magical arts of Circe and Calypso, an ordinary, mortal woman, is perhaps one of the first true feminists in history who will pay the price of their deeds and words with their lives. Antigone opposes the violent tyranny but is a continuous source of love: she accompanies her father, Oedipus, old and blind, to the end of his existence and then, always out of love, she gives her dead brother a final embrace and farewell.

Some historians define the rituals of cleansing the corpse, the last farewell, and the birth of burial as the beginning of Western civilization. Here, Antigone stands up to savage nature and acts spontaneously without receiving any help or compassion. Even Achilles was moved by Priam's requests to bury Hector, whom he killed, granting his father a dignified burial for his son. Achilles was a warrior, not a tyrant. Marshall also identifies the "celebration" of loss, the right of mourning, a human right, going beyond the stereotypes that people want to share only victorious events. The mourning of the loss is embedded in our human being, and it is a violent action to take away this important ritual. The etymology of the word loss differs in many countries: in English, it comes from "destruction," of Germanic origin; related to Old Norse *los*, "breaking up of the ranks of an army" and "loose." In Italian, French, Spanish and Portuguese, it comes from Latin, *"Perdere"*, Latin etymon from *Para* and *Dare,* "Give Against," in the opposite sense, destroy, dissipate. So, if there is a breakdown in the Norse culture in the ranks, there is a straight confrontation with something frontal. This something frontal can be a disease, a war, a battle, a match, a competition, or a dispute. So, there is no loss without something essential for us to stake: the lives of our brothers and remembering them with funerary tributes in case of death.

Antigone's end is tragic. Creon orders her to be walled up alive in a cave, while Ismene continues her existence as peacefully as the river near Thebes.

CREON
And yet, wert bold enough to break the law?
ANTIGONE
Yea, for these laws were not ordained of Zeus,
And she who sits enthroned with gods below,
Justice, enacted, not these human laws.
Nor did I deem that thou, a mortal man,
Could'st by a breath annul and override
The immutable unwritten laws of Heaven.
They were not born today nor yesterday;
They die not; and none knoweth whence they sprang.
I was not like, who feared no mortal's frown,
To disobey these laws and so provoke
The wrath of Heaven. I knew that I must die,
E'en hadst thou not proclaimed it; and if death
Is thereby hastened, I shall count it gain.
For death is gain to him whose life, like mine,
Is full of misery. Thus my lot appears
Not sad, but blissful; for had I endured
To leave my mother's son unburied there,
I should have grieved with reason, but not now.

The burial funeral is a ritual that goes back to the roots of our history, claiming, as Sophocles wrote, that not doing violates Divine Laws, not humble human laws.

And let us come to today's events, the tyrant is there! Or at least the tyranny is far more extensive than in the city of Thebes, and in Ukraine, the dead of both factions are left unburied. Although it is not clear who is responsible for killing whom, the corpses are sometimes vandalized and placed on display in ordinary places, such as in front of supermarkets, with the express mandate to frighten, incite terror, and break the oldest laws, those related to honoring the dead. The escalation we are experiencing is daily, which will undoubtedly have tragic repercussions on the war's outcome. It's hard to believe, but tragedy lies, not just in ancient literature, but also in our daily lives.

Another story, partially analogous, is the issue of burials in times of COVID-19 (and it is now four years, 2020, 2021, 2022, and 2023, so it will be good that some rules may change). It is worth mentioning the pain and sadness of what happened in 2020, where funeral rites were not celebrated at all, and the bodies were cremated, without the ashes being returned to their loved ones. Indeed, the fate of the Covid-19 dead during the first wave's carnage in the middle of the lockdown was uncertain. In those terrible days, many websites opened for those who remained to write about the memory of their dead, and it was the only surrogate way to cope with all this sudden death.

Here from the website *memorie.it,* a letter to a deceased mother, after one year when she passed away:

> *Dear Mum. It has been a year. We miss you. We miss your smile and your unforgettable, beautiful blue eyes. We miss you. We were not ready. Of course, life takes its course. But the epidemic did the rest: emergency and distance distorted the normality of death. And to lose you like this is even more challenging to accept. We want the memory to bring back the sweetest memories, those that soften the heart and transform anguish into nostalgia and hope, capable of restarting in the knowledge that you are still very close to us, an integral part of the world.*
>
> *You are here, and we will find you again in the values you believed in the most and passed on to your children, in the poems you still recited in your own way, in your land overlooking the lake, in the daisies and pink flowers that amazed you every spring; in the sea you loved so much; in the music that made you happy; in the memory of your last walks when, as a child again, you were filled with joy as you perceived a whole new world in a world that was the same as ever. You are here in the thousands of fragments of life that each one of us will treasure forever. You are also here in the simple little things you had prepared with infinite tenderness for the farewell: the envelopes you drew for us, your photo, and the poem from daddy you wanted to take with you forever.*

This was a letter written after one year of grief. Still, suppose we access this website and read the lines of memorials written in March and April 2020. In that case, we are not only invested in sorrow, but the most dominant emotion expressed, anger:

> *They could not safeguard you, they have forbidden me to see you, and when you went away, I was not there holding your hand, and you were scared, and probably you also asked yourself, why nobody was there with you.*

When death is forecasted, one can somehow "get prepared," even if it is so violent in nature, to think about the legacy, processing the mourning, but here, and I underline especially in Lombardy where in the first wave we had the highest peak of mortality in Bergamo, that nobody was ready, neither the citizens and family members nor the health care professionals.

The healthcare professionals were overwhelmed physically and psychologically by the sudden outbreak. They needed to bring their ceremonials to the deeds: some wrote bullet point lists of the names of the disappeared people (among them colleagues), some stood in silence for a long time, and some broke this silence, putting the down in black and white. How? Using narrative tools. Here, two short stories written by doctors in Bergamo are reported as an example of processing loss, a figurative funeral and act of rebellion, analogous to the way in which Polynices' burial was legally impossible at that time.

> *Outside the sirens, inside the silence*
>
> *Losing shoes in the ER is not uncommon, but they are usually immediately claimed by the owner, his relatives, the ward, or promptly returned by the ER staff.*
>
> *That night, however, was different; the shoe was abandoned in the corner for the entire ten hours of my shift. On the way home, I found myself thinking about its owner, that elegant man in his fifties who had been lying on a stretcher for a long time, wondering if fate had chosen to turn him into a number, pushed through the long-deserted corridors of the hospital to his room, in the respectful silence of illness, with the loneliness of the plague victim.*

The presence of a family member or an acquaintance would have been enough to realize that the shoe was missing immediately. Still, this terrible epidemic has made us lonely in every situation. Alone in waiting for the judgment of the disease, alone in suffering, alone in the quarantines of our homes. Alone in having to take care of ourselves even when ill, no one to check that our shoes are both in place.

Another way of processing the violence of the sudden immense death wave was in the novel written by a doctor, still from Bergamo, of a man who lost his spouse.

Montalbano does not solve all cases.

Stairs, at my age, hurt. My ankles swell, and I feel intense cramps in my calves. Today it was sunny, it was April, and in the garden, I put the first tomatoes., Fabiola's favorite. I have not been out of the house for two months; I haven't met anyone for two months, and, living in the countryside, only the rabbits' scampering and the rooster's crowing keep me company. Sitting at the table, I am peeling an apple. I spread a cloth to avoid getting dirty, and the potatoes are cooked in the oven. I look out the window at my vegetable garden. It is pretty, tidy, divided by crops. The little wall that separates it from the garage is now in place; I've been working on it with splinters. I sigh contentedly and close the shutters. The light from the oven sucks me in and switches off my brain. I see Fabiola, our nights. Before the shelter, two nights before, she surprised me.

We were in the bedroom, and Montalbano was playing on the TV. "We are old Richi" is what she called me when we were alone, Riccardo in front of the others. I did not answer her, frowning in disagreement. 'We're just less young. What do we lack? Nothing," I tried to shut her up. "Time, Richi, we lack time." He turned away with his hands clasped under his pillow. I looked at the blanket and was enchanted. Since I was no longer working, I appreciated the little things. She had embroidered a patchwork of sunflowers along the edges by hand. I spread my beard with my fingers and looked at her shoulders. She was breathing differently. Montalbano was about to solve the case, but I needed to pay attention. "Are you asleep?" I asked her.

No, I do not sleep'. "I'm not sleepy, Fabi". "You're never sleepy; it's old age. You sleep too much in the afternoon." I ran my palm over the sheet to flatten a crease, but all I did was move it further down. Fabi's feet were cold; I could feel them on mine. "You, the vegetable garden and the maintenance. Why don't we resume with the trips?" "They cost too much." What a stupid answer I gave her. We were not sailing in gold, but our pensions were enough—we could have afforded a trip to Porto Empedocle. Fabiola snorted. She folded her legs and ran her hand through her hair. On her bedside table, the rosary hung from the abat-jour. She had bought it in Rome.

'Luca has made quite a family,' she said. Luca is our son. "He is happy." She took the silver frame she held next to the rosary in her hands. "I'm so proud." "You are a grandmother." "Don't remind me you're old." I smiled at her. Our gazes did not change with the years. We were as much in love as we were in our twenties under the ice cream man's porch complaining about the rain. Advertising. They were offering women's underwear. Fabi sat with her pillow behind her back. She crinkled her eyes and yawned. Her voice still relaxed from yawning, she said, 'Good times when I could wear them.

I didn't want to, but I burst out laughing. I laughed with gusto, leaning forward from laughter and sobs.

"What are you laughing at?" "You never wore them." "Are you kidding?" "When never?" "When you weren't there." I looked up at the ceiling. She lay back down. She was breathing differently.

The timer went off, and I recovered from the memories. The red peel unrolls on the cloth. The potatoes are ready. I take them out of the oven. In the living room, the phone rings, it is Luca. I answer as I run my hand over my calves. He asks how I am if I have cooked or made the bed and taken the pills; I reassure him. Since Fabiola is no longer here, Montalbano makes me melancholy. [1]

But this was the horrific 2020, which has no comparison to the current knowledge of this disease. Was it legal to abolish the funerals in 2020? Yes, it was legal, and it was, for sure, the outcome of the cost-benefit analysis for the majority. However, the downsides of this decision are still evident after two years in the memories of citizens. Moreover, for those who survived the carnage were left to cope for longer than would have they been able to say "goodbye" through authentic rituals, religious or layman.

4.1 The Funeral Rituals

Anthropologists have had the opportunity to study funeral rituals closely in different corners of the world and analyse them from various perspectives. One of the most famous scholars and theorists in this field was Arnold Van Gennep [2] who more than half a century ago theorized that the so-called "rites of passage", are still an essential element in the anthropological study of rituals today. Under this name, Van Gennep enclosed all those rituals that mark critical moments of course from one status to another in the individual's life: birth, the path from puberty to adulthood, marriage and death. The most valuable contribution to this anthropologist's studies is the theory on the existence of a liminal phase dictated by the ritual itself. In this phase, the individual is no longer in the state he is leaving behind, nor even in the one he is heading towards; instead, he can be said to be in the *limen* (from the Latin: "threshold" or "boundary") between the two. During this transitional phase, ordinary life is momentarily suspended, and the individual prepares to be socially ready for his new status and social existence. It is a moment of transition, in which the separation from what one had already taken place, while the incorporation into what one is about to witness has not yet taken shape.

Funerals extend this journey to the other world in a series of transition rites and help structure the mourning process of survivors. Transition, rather than separation, is singled out as the predominating element of funerary rites, affecting both the living and the dead, outlining the potential dangers for each as ritual changes in identity occur. Yet, almost as a law of life, these changes also affect the renewal of much-needed energy. One ignored element in Van Gennep's work concerns fear of funerals may be the result of "defensive procedures," protecting against departed souls or the "contagion of death" and helping to "dispose of eternal enemies" of the survivors.

We hoped for the disappearance of the virus. Instead, while writing (August 2022), the Omicron Beta 5 now has supremacy over all the different variants, and yes, it is a VOC, a variable of concern. Unfortunately, the mortality rate in Italy in July 2022 is still high: 176 deaths in one day because of the virus. Coming to the burial rituals, I just recently discovered that the relatives of those who passed due to COVID-19 (I do not wish to enter into the conundrum of the classification of dying *with Covid or of Covid*, on which still three years of scientific debate were not able to prevail on political use of the virus, but I would like to see more up-to-date data from the section of the Istituto Superiore di Sanità, whose mortality data presenting

4.1 The Funeral Rituals

age, gender, and concomitant diseases are ended in January 2022) receive the coffin already sealed, without having the possibility of seeing the body, carrying, for instance, the favorite earrings to the beloved. I think of my death, I know which earrings I wish to burn with me, as I know which ring I have chosen to take away. Whereas for the other non-Covid related deaths, the last salutation is possible since the corps belongs to a privileged situation of deaths and, therefore can be touched by loved ones.

Today's thanatologists, experts on death (from the Greek word "Thanatos" meaning death) as it relates to a variety of competencies such as, counseling, psychotherapy, activism, palliative care, and healthcare, are trying to help relatives to cope with this violent Burial, that denies the possibility to see their dearests. In the mourning therapy group, they ask to carry some personal items of the person who passed away, the identical things that they would have been loving to give to those in this ritual of passage, on the threshold, to bring with them in the last departure. This practice promotes soothing and consolatory creativity to counteract the anger and soften emotions.

"Departures" (Japanese: おくりびと, Hepburn: *Okuribito,* "the one who sends away") is a 2008 Japanese film about a young man who returns to his hometown after a failed career as a cellist and comes across a job as a *nōkanshi*, the traditional Japanese funeral rite of preparing dead bodies for burial. In Japan, this profession is highly stigmatised, thus he is ashamed to tell his circle of relatives and friends what he does. In other words, he is a "thanato-aesthetics", who is responsible for alleviating the fears of relatives through the beautification of the corpse. As they see their loved ones, thoughtfully adorned with makeup, jewels, and perfumes, they are able to reframe their thoughts to see that their loved one is not dead, but merely "sleeping." With time the main protagonist realizes that his prior experiences as a cellist have granted him a special ability to handle the bodies with incomparable delicacy and tenderness, hence making him a masterful *nokanshi.* In the end, it is through this sacred art that enable him to reconcile with his father, whose body he must prepare for burial.

This film reinforces the importance of caring for the people who have recently passed away in their respective "ecosystem" of people, objects, and symbols. In addition to the *nokasnhi*, the *Antigons* were tasked with washing the bodies and caressing the faces of the dead. We all need to say goodbye to our loved ones before their last journey, by seeing their bodies, carefully dressed, and made up. To illustrate this point further, I quote an Italian film that was released in 2021 titled "It was the Hand of God," directed by Paolo Sorrentino, Oscar winner for "The Great Beauty." The film was produced in honor of the deaths of both his parents, for an accident, when he was only a teenager.

The actor who plays the role of the young Sorrentino cries repeatedly, "they didn't let me see them", with "They" referring to the healthcare workers and the coroner. Is it not an act of violence, sealing the coffin and denying the intimacy of the last farewell?

We, family members, are also called, like Antigone, to be there in a complete way in the last vision, the preamble to the final farewell. The sealed coffin is an additional loss, adding to the actual grief. Can we prudently afford to change the rules? Or at least to let the loved ones choose whether they want to see, with their own eyes and for the last time, the body of the one they loved? Of course, it is an ethical dilemma, between love, mourning, and safety. However, there is an auto determination principle, that risks being violated by the standardization and over-simplification of the whole procedure outlining the management of the bodies of those who passed of COVID-19 or other deadly transmissible infectious diseases. But with safe care, just as productivity cannot be stopped, there is a need to stand as witnesses before the open coffin.

"Thanatos" in his brutality is possibly the most violent thing to exist on earth as Hesiod states [3] in his Theogony:

Have the houses here of the turbid night the children
   Death and Sleep terrible Gods; and never the glittering Sun
   with his rays does he behold them, nor when he ascends
   Heaven, nor when down from heaven he descends. Of these,
   Above the earth the one mild Sleep flies on the sea's infinite back
   and have a heart of honey for all;
   Of iron has the other his heart of bronze implacable
   His soul sits; and when once a mortal is seized
   He leaves him no more; and even the Immortals hate him. (Hesiod, Theogony, vv. 758–766)

Too absurd, mysterious, difficult, if not impossible to accept is *Thanatos*: rituals of interconnection among realms of death and life and people are the best remedy for the others who remain here, with their lives in their hand (Fig. 4.1)

Fig. 4.1 Gold will fall (photo by Maria Giulia Marini)

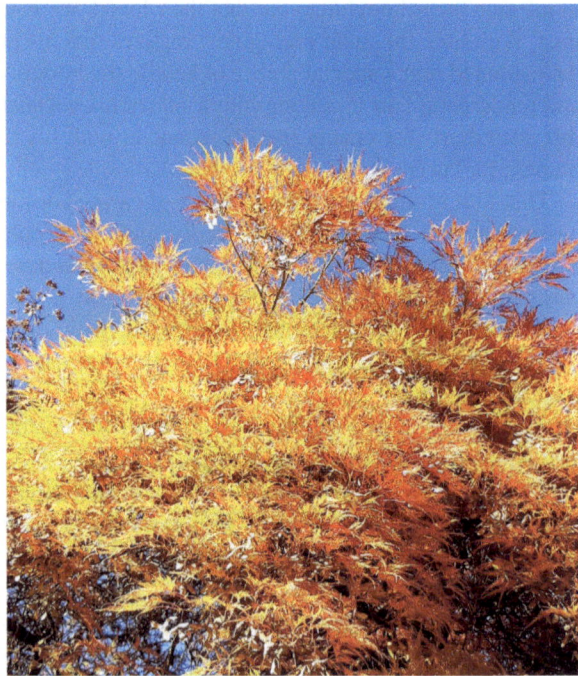

4.2 Practice Time

One art (Elisabeth Bishop)
>The art of losing isn't hard to master
>so many things seem filled with the intent
>to be lost that their loss is no disaster.
>Lose something every day. Accept the fluster
>of lost door keys, the hour badly spent.
>The art of losing isn't hard to master.
>Then practice losing farther, losing faster:
>places, and names, and where it was you meant
>to travel. None of these will bring disaster.
>I lost my mother's watch. And look! my last, or
>next-to-last, of three loved houses went.
>The art of losing isn't hard to master.
>I lost two cities, lovely ones. And, vaster,
>some realms I owned, two rivers, a continent.
>I miss them, but it wasn't a disaster.
>—Even losing you (the joking voice, a gesture
>I love) I shan't have lied. It's evident
>the art of losing's not too hard to master
>though it may look like (*Write* it!) like disaster.

This poem composed by Elizabeth Bishop, winner of the Pulitzer Prize in Poetry in 1956 [4].

She has always been ill, confronted by a loss of health, family boundaries, and years of life.

Now think to her words and analyse the language. What inspires you? Regarding your professional career, do you think you lost something, and how did you cope with this sense of loss?

In our illness plot, narrative space for patients and caregivers, and parallel chart, narrative spaces for healthcare providers, at ISTUD, we many times put this prompt for reflective writing…

I lost/ I earned…

4.2.1 Losing a Patient for a Surgeon [5]

Surgery is a branch of medicine which is associated not only with the touching of the body, but to the entering in the body, dissecting it, resecting, using surgical tools such as lancet, cutters, and more. More sophisticated are the "hands of the surgeon" today (the etymology of the word "surgery" has its origins in ancient Greek. It comes from the word *Xheir,* meaning "hand", translated into the Italian word *Chirurgia,* where the last suffix, comes as well from ancient Greek from *ergon,* and means "work" and in English it this *Xheir-* comes Sur- and then *ergon, -gery*), helped by artificial intelligence which allows for the execution of masterpieces of microsurgeries. Undergoing a surgery can be a matter of lifesaving or a routine intervention for a patient. Not to mention, the numerous publications about the fears of the anesthesia, "the missing reawakening" or of a very unlikely surgeon's error. Surgery can be "a violent" landscape characterized by blood and flesh, with surgical instruments, scissors, drills, spreaders, curettes, spoon bones. All these images contribute to the creation of the archetype of "painful" medicine, especially before the revolutionary discovery of anesthesia.

However, too little is known about the emotions felt by surgeons who have lost a patient. They are too often labeled as detached— anesthetized of emotions. Now, we will change this short-sighted belief.

Losing a patient is an experience that all surgeons are likely to face at some point in their careers. The circumstances surrounding these deaths differ—one patient's life might have been in the process of ending for years due to a terminal illness, meanwhile another might suffer complications during what should be a routine procedure. These events can be devastating for everyone involved, and with that in mind, several Fellows of the American College of Surgeons (ACS) share strategies they have learned that ease the difficulty of patient loss, as well as advice they would offer to people considering careers in surgery.

Geoffrey P. Dunn [6] MD, General Surgeon within the Department of Surgery, and Medical Director, operating also in the Palliative Care Consultation Service at the University of Pittsburgh Medical Center (UPMC) said he has seen a change in how death is perceived in the surgical world. Dunn discusses how when he started his career 30 years ago, surgeons were not inclined to see death as a natural occurrence. The main question was, "Is my treatment of the patient working?" Recently, however, Dunn has noticed the focus shift from a single instance of death to improving the surgeon's ability to anticipate it and to enhance the patient's comfort level during this time.

When he began practicing, Dunn learned how important it is to be completely honest with patients' families because, many times, he knew the families and would often cross paths with them outside of the hospital. And as the son, grandson, and great-grandson of surgeons who practiced at the same institution, Dr. Dunn confessed he felt a great responsibility to his patients and their loved ones. Recently, he treated a 102-year-old man on whom his grandfather also had operated.

Dunn states that connection can be helpful, but it can also make it more painful if something happens to the patient. Even in those circumstances, though, staying in touch with the patient's family has helped him to cope. One of the first losses Dr. Dunn experienced was with a patient on whom his father had operated years before. After the funeral, the family invited him to dinner, where he heard them talk about the man's life. He and the family kept in touch for years.

He also became an early believer in *the value of a condolence letter* (an exquisite example of "Intelligent Kindness," soothing the violence caused by a force of nature), which serves as a tribute to the patient and a source of comfort to the survivors. In those letters, he makes sure to recall the qualities of the patient and offers a way to stay connected: *"Death is not a final, defining point for the individual or the relationship that occurred around it"*.

Developing a relationship with a patient's family also helped Dr. Danielle Saunders Walsh, a Pediatric Surgeon, get through the loss of a patient. She said the death of every child affects her, regardless of how well she knows the family: *"Children bring a different perspective in dealing with death. In general, we view them as innocent. We see it as a loss of an opportunity for someone to experience a full life"*.

One of her first experiences with loss occurred with a teenage patient with a congenital disability that became increasingly problematic as the girl matured. The girl died suddenly while she was performing a procedure. Losing this patient was tough, and she contemplated whether a career in surgery was right for her. *"If this is so painful, why am I doing it?"* she wondered. But at the funeral, the girl's mother told her, '*I hope you don't give up,*'" which reassured her that she should continue her chosen career.

Many conversations with patients and families would be more effortless if all Western societies could view death as a natural part of life, no matter how brief or lengthy that life may be. But we have yet to quit there as a society because people tend to think there is always more, medically, that can be done to fix the situation. Our Western Kantian imperative: fix it.

Patricia J. Numann, MD, is a distinguished Teaching Professor Emeritus at State University of New York. She has noticed that accepting patients' death seems harder now than when she started her career as a surgeon. When she was a medical student in the 1960s at the State University, there were no intensive care units and *"A lot more people died. [They] didn't have these extraordinary, heroic things we could do for people."*

At that time, she was always reasonably comfortable talking about death. As a child, she would walk around Woodlawn Cemetery in the Bronx, NY, with her aunt, and they would look at the flowers on the graves. As a third-year medical student, Dr. Numann left school to help care for her mother, who had pancreatic cancer and wanted to spend her remaining time at home. Her mother died after she returned to school. Her mother was, in a way, the first patient she lost.

From that experience, she saw that some patients cling to life, waiting for certain events—babies to be born, graduations, weddings, etc.—before they pass away. She said it can be important to the process that they have something to look forward to, and she always made it a habit to visit dying patients at home when she could. Many families want to know that their loved ones are not alone when they are close to death. Family members have asked her to sit with patients if they are not emotionally strong enough in the moment.

She would always try to go to the family's calling hours after the death of a patient to cope. Dr. Numann added that many people do not realize how much surgeons miss some of the patients they have treated: *"Some patients become like part of your extended family as part of a trusted relationship; they would get to know what was going on in each other's lives"*.

In the last two years, I was involved in the Congress Initiative, "The surgeon as a humanist" [7]. After speaking with surgeons from Italy, Spain and the US, I think that they are among the specialists who though are often stereotyped as cold, stiff, and not in touch with their emotions, are changing the paradigms of medicine by introducing extraordinary courses that pull back the curtains concealing the immense joy surrounding promising interventions and lives saved, as well as the grief experienced due to the catastrophic events that have occurred within the last few years.

4.2.2 The Loss of a Patient from the Perspective of a Nurse [8]

Nurses spend around 86% of their time with their patients. From a patient's perspective, "care times," defined as time with at least one healthcare worker of a designated type in their intensive care unit room, are distributed as follows: 13.11% with physicians, 86.14% with nurses, and 8.14% with critical support staff (i.e., respiratory therapists, pharmacists, etc.) [9]:

On top of this objective time measurement, physicians, like consultants, are sometimes feared by patients; since they are highly educated, they play higher roles in healthcare organizations, often in a hierarchy. In my experience assessing the narratives of patients and fragments of their biographies, I have consistently noticed that this vulnerability (the narrative side of patients) is most often cared for and encouraged by nurses, hence why I call their practice "narrative nursing," to add another label to this ecosystem. They see all the family members, not only one caregiver, but also the siblings, grandchildren, children, and friends. For them, dealing with a patient's death is losing someone they know—someone they regularly talk to, joke with, and have built an intimate relationship with.

From the narrative of a nurse:

> *I honestly think the most stressful and emotionally taxing part of dealing with patient death is being there for their families, which is very important. I honestly feel like we do not get enough education or practice with this part because we are there for treatment, and I know how to care for patients. I know what to do to save them. But when we cannot save them, what comes after that is dealing with the family while they say goodbye to their loved one. We are there with them afterwards while they are grieving. That is the hardest thing for me in my career.*
>
> *It was the hardest thing for me to get used to from the beginning, and I always thought the actual scenario of trying to save somebody or their passing away would be the hardest. For me, it is the emotional part of dealing with the remaining family members who are grieving and so upset. I think a lot of that is because I'm very empathetic. I have always been that way.*
>
> *.... My advice in dealing with the families is that it is okay to be silent. I always used to feel like I needed to say something when a tragic situation was happening. I was in the room with a family who was saying bye to their dead loved one, and I felt like I should be saying something or talking to them, trying to console them, but there's nothing you can say to help them. There's nothing you can say to take their pain away. Sometimes, just being there, handing out tissues, trying to hand out water, or anything you can just to make them a little more comfortable is all you can do.*

> *Sometimes, people just need a hug. Not everybody is a hugger, but sometimes family members want you to be there with them. Sometimes, they need a hug, a shoulder to cry on, and you can be that person. You don't always need to be saying something.*
>
> *There is no correct answer here; all you can do is what feels right. Often for me, I found that that was silence and waiting for them to start talking. When they speak and initiate and want to talk more about what's happening, I'm there, and I'll talk to them as well.*
>
> *A second thing I would say is, please try not to blame yourself and try and find something wrong with what you did when somebody dies in your care. We've tried everything we can to save somebody. Their body couldn't handle it, and it was just time for them to go, even though it doesn't feel like it's time and doesn't feel like it's right. There's too much, too many factors going on, so try not to blame yourself, try not to replay scenarios repeatedly in your head blaming yourself.*

Other fragments of nurses' voices while talking to the deceased to "*... bid him farewell, wishing him a safe journey ... telling him he did good in this world*".

> *Although there is no life, you must care for your patient in many ways: psychologically, physically, emotionally .... Although there is no life, the body, and those parts [nursing care] you still have to go through.*

Self-compassion is the first key for nurses to stop blaming themselves, and this ruminant thinking is an act of self-administered violence. The second key that must be given to open the shut doors of our Western society is stopping considering human beings as immortal gods. We might learn so much from the Buddhist concept of impermanence; once we acknowledge this reality, grief could become less hard.

Above are authentic narratives from surgeons and nurses about their loss of a patient. What can you bring home from these witnesses? What would you add as other coping factors, if any? And how might you try to apply the concept of impermanent, or "the art of losing"?

References

1. Voci da una comunità narrante Il fiocco viola—Bergamo, il Covid, una ferita collettiva. Durango Edizioni; 2021
2. Van Gennep A. The rites of passage. University of Chicago Press; 2019.
3. Hesiods. Work and days; n.d.
4. Elizabeth Bishop. One art. The Newyorker; 1976.
5. https://bulletin.facs.org/2015/02/patient-loss-surgeons-describe-how-they-cope/. n.d.
6. Dunn GP. Surgery, palliative care, and the American College of Surgeons. Ann Palliative Med. 2015;
7. Jonatham Mc Farland, Susana Magalhaes. Congress in Porto, Porto; 2022.
8. https://www.medpagetoday.com/publichealthpolicy/generalprofessionalissues/8486; n.d.
9. Butler R, Monsalve M, Thomas GW, Herman T, Segre AM, Polgreen PM, Suneja M. Estimating time physicians and other health care workers spend with patients in an intensive care unit using a sensor network. Am J Med. 2018;131(8):972.e9–972.e15

Chapter 5
Communication in Case of Isolation: The Tribute to the Young People, Distance Learning, Hikikomori and Anorexia Cases

Because I could not stop for Death—
He kindly stopped for me—
The Carriage held but just Ourselves—
And Immortality.
We slowly drove—He knew no haste
And I had put away
My labor and my leisure, too,
For His Civility—
We passed the school, where Children strove
At Recess—in the Ring—
We passed the Fields of Gazing Grain—
We passed the Setting Sun—
Or rather—He passed us—
The Dews drew quivering and chill—
For only Gossamer, my Gown—
My Tippet—only Tulle—
We paused before a House that seemed
A Swelling of the Ground—
The Roof was scarcely visible—
The Cornice—in the Ground—
Since then—'tis Centuries—and yet
Feels shorter than the day
I first surmised the Horses' Heads
Were toward Eternity—

This poem is of the first Hikikomori poet in modern literature: Emily Dickinson. After closely examining the biography of Emily Dickinson, one of the greatest poetesses to write about Life, Death and Immortality, the Contemplation of Nature, and

© The Author(s), under exclusive license to Springer Nature
Switzerland AG 2024
M. G. Marini, *Non-violent Communication and Narrative Medicine for Promoting Sustainable Health*, New Paradigms in Healthcare,
https://doi.org/10.1007/978-3-031-58691-0_5

about the suffering she endured in such a sophisticated and ironic way, we discover that she was affected by Hikikomori. This mental illness, which was first identified in Japan, is characterized by a "pulling inward," or willful social isolation. The poetess spent a great deal of her life closed in her room, avoiding contact with the external world.

She was born in Amherst and received her education at Amherst Academy in Massachusetts. Though the reasons for Dickinson's final departure from the academy in 1848 are unknown, theories say that her fragile emotional state may have played a role and/or that her father decided to pull her from the school. She left college when she was a teenager and asked permission from her father to do something that typical of those with Hikikomori, that is, to stay up during the middle of the night, (from 3 am to 5am) to compose poems, (though Hikikomori today commonly play with video games during these hours) and to sleep during the day. She displayed the same symptoms, namely a low sense of self-worth, that the Hikikomori youth has. It's such a shame that Dickinson did not believe she was beautiful nor witty enough, and as a result prepared for life to quit her family and launch herself in the possibility of building her new family.

The astonishing thing is that she lived more than 30 years in this condition, until the age of 56, which is very uncommon given the state of her health and the life expectancy of the time period.

To be more specific, she also suffered from a kidney disease that brought her some seizures, loss of consciousness, and pain. She was surrounded by a lovely and, at the same time, mysterious family. Her mother suffered from bouts of depression, and her father was a follower of illuminism, trying to move on from Puritan teachings and ideologies, however with a very straightforward and harsh character, her brother was a dubious man with an official wife and a semi-official lover.

Her sister Lavinia was the only "caregiver" who challenged her choice of isolation, her vision of life and death, and her values—Emily the utmost introverted, Lavinia the utmost extroverted. Lavinia is the person to whom Emily was and should be still now, in her immortal verse, the most grateful. Her sister stood by her side during her difficult life and believed in her talent, although no one around praised her innovative poetry. She published more than sixteen hundred poems, most without a title. In her life, the poetess had the misfortune to see only seven of her poems published, and she was considered quite controversial by the critics of that period, labelling her as the poetess of unhappiness.

Indeed, she was very sensible and touched by the deaths of people close to her family and within her family, many of her works were influenced by the outbreak of the American Civil War, with blood spilled between North and South daily. Emily could not stand all this death. Her loneliness prompted her to find shelter in love, mainly through love letters. Still, she kept falling in love with the wrong men, either married men (reverends) or not inaccessible ones, showing, in my opinion, the unconscious willingness to suffer for the sake of unrequited love.

However, living in her parallel world, she was able to build, despite all her pain and fear of inadequacy, an intense world of faith, which goes far beyond the traditional Puritan sermons of that age. She was able to find the spirituality in Nature, the extraordinary in the ordinary, giving up the lace and embroideries in exchange for dressing only white clothes, just like her verses: clean and dry with no decoration.

To make a prairie it takes a clover and one bee,
One clover, and a bee.
And revery.
The revery alone will do,
If bees are few

Simple, so very advanced in her style, fragmented, that anticipates the modern way of being a poet: she profoundly influenced the direction of 20th-century poetry.

5.1 The Violence of Social Pressure

A culture of over-competitiveness triggers violence in youth and creates an "us" against "them" [1], and social pressure creates expectations which, if already hard to handle for adults, are sometimes almost impossible for young people to bear.

I'm Nobody! Who are you? Are you—Nobody—too?
Then there's a pair of us!
Don't tell! They'd advertise—you know!
How dreary—to be—Somebody!
How public—like a Frog—
To tell one's name—the livelong June—
To an admiring Bog!

Being Nobody is better than being a croaking frog in a pond. It has some advantages: escapes from the demanding and challenging and annoying things to appear, to have a reputation to safeguard, to become successful, to become famous, as social media requires from us.

Youth affected by the Hikikomori syndrome is the expression, the dramatic dissent to of the disease of our society, in which one must be famous, rich, and beautiful. Dickinson teaches us that sometimes *being Nobody* gives us the possibility of a happier life and to continue the parade of the Frog, which boisterously assigns names and roles to everybody. However, we might develop illness, being stuck in the same room.

In a recent study [2], researchers found out that in the Hikikomori group, the level of HDL (the good cholesterol) is lower than in active students, which they call a "prognostic factor". It is quite known in the scientific literature that HDL arises when people practice active sports, which is not included in the Hikikomori profile. Therefore, a low level of HDL might be considered a risk factor for becoming a withdrawal from the world. Emily also should have had a very low level of HDL, since she barely left her room and ate her meals at her desk, where she wrote.

Emily published only seven poems during her lifetime. She did have the ambition to become famous anyway; she wrote because, for her, it was therapeutic, much in the same way Virginia Woolf did. She had applied narrative medicine while writing without knowing it. For example, carefully observed the way she describes her epileptic seizure:

I felt a Funeral, in my brain,
And Mourners to and fro
Kept treading – treading – till it seemed
That Sense was breaking through –
And when they all were seated,
A Service, like a Drum –
Kept beating – beating – till I thought
My mind was going numb –
And then I heard them lift a Box
And creak across my Soul
With those same Boots of Lead, again,
Then space – began to toll,
As all the Heavens were a Bell,
And Being, but an Ear,
And I, and Silence, some strange Race,
Wrecked, solitary, here
And then a Plank in Reason, broke,
And I dropped down, and down –
And hit a World, at every plunge,
And Finished knowing – then –

Impressive, the clues that she gives us to understand Epilepsy. The reader may deduce that for Dickinson, the rational mind was a real value against the short-sightedness of religiosity, to have a "momentary eclipse of reason" was like to have a funeral of her brain.

Narrative medicine is not a new invention, but rather, anyone who has ever written about their illness—or told, composed music, painted, or sculpted a representation of it— whatever they did, they transformed the untold illness into something marvelous through narrative medicine, a heritage of humankind.

5.1.1 The Forced Hikikomori Youth Lockdown

The lockdown of hundreds of millions of young people in 2020 and partly in 2021, and still, in an on-and-off way, in 2022 at schools, isolation somehow recreated, even with a social good aim, conditions in which Hikikomori syndrome could flourish.

In Italy, for instance, empirical data described an increase in the use of digital media near bedtime during the lockdown [3]. Another critical point was the expected increase of new technology-dependent habits during the COVID-19 pandemic that may persist in the aftermath, such as online shopping, food delivery, online education courses, exclusively online social interaction, and online medical and psychological appointments.

Such life habits may be associated with *hikikomori* cases and could increase their prevalence soon. The rise in the prevalence of psychiatric symptoms and disorders also may result in more *hikikomori* cases. Studies from China highlighted a substantial increase in anxiety and depression [4]. During the COVID-19 outbreak, with a depression prevalence of 43.7% among Chinese adolescents [5].

Later, we will come back to make additional comments on the narrative health status of the young people and how to communicate with them, but now...

Were almost 3 years of isolation for the youth damaging?

Despite fearing real life in the outside world, Dickinson possesses a powerful set of inner resource, such as the ability to re-invent her language of expression. What about today's generation of teenagers? Youth health surveys have been conducted in Finland, the USA, France, the UK and Italy during the pandemic. An increase in domestic accidents and head injuries due to suspected abuse or violence was reported. In addition, health-related behaviors also worsened: more time spent in front of the PC and on social media (from 2.9 h up to 5.1 on average per day) and a significant reduction in the level of physical activity (up to 64%). Finally, sleep disturbances and increased consumption of "junk food" were reported.

All studies reported significant variations in the quality and quantity of sleep for all age groups, a decrease in the length of night rest in preschool and school-age children, and 63.9% of adolescents reported sleeping for less than 8 h a night. 61% of children and adolescents (mean age 10.4 years; range 6–14 years) reported difficulty falling asleep and fragmented sleep. Regarding the consumption of less healthy food, studies conducted in Italy, Spain, and India reported an overall increase in food consumption in 57.3% of young Italians (age 6–14 years), with significant increases in the consumption of crisps, red meat, and sugary drinks ($p < 0.005$), and reduced consumption of fruit and vegetables ($p < 0.001$), especially among adolescents [6]. In May 2020, during the COVID-19 pandemic, ED visits for suspected suicide attempts began to increase among adolescents aged 12–17 years, especially among girls. During February 2020 and March 2021, ED visits for suspected suicide attempts were 50.6% higher among girls aged 12–17 than during the same period in 2019; among boys aged 12–17, ED visits for suspected suicide attempts increased by 3.7%.

It is difficult to collect youth voices outside social networks. There were many clamors from all COVID-19- patients, but teenagers were somehow silenced. However, social networks are more used to give a "perfect" image of the self than to show the true face behind the mask.

In his account on illness *At the Will of the Body*, Arthur Frank wrote, "...for the times I have had to keep silent and for those who are still silent." The historical lack of traditional texts and the continuing need for appropriate clinical environments for adolescents testifies to the silence surrounding this population's medical, social, and literary needs.

A group of scholars from ISTUD's Master in Applied Narrative Medicine program collected the voices of teens to gain a deeper understanding of what happened during school hours while they were distance learning at home. Here is the narrative plot proposed to the students:

I, before the pandemic....
Then the pandemic came...
Covid was...
Studying was...
Now...
Studying...
With my friends...
For the future...

This plot was developed based on two assumptions: the diachronic movement, which is helpful to invite people to look forward into the future, and the Natural Semantic Metalanguage. Anna Wierzbicka, Professor of Linguistics and Founder of the Natural Semantic Metalanguage (NSM) approach (together with Cliff Goddard) provided a revolutionary perspective on language (Goddard and Wierzbicka, 2002). NSM is based on empirical evidence that all languages share 65 simple core words (the 'primes' or atoms of meaning). Using English words (since this essay is written in English), let us briefly spell out some of these semantic building blocks are: "before", "now", "moment", "after", "feel," "think", "say", "do", "know", "happen", "hear", "see", "touch", "want", "do not want", "big", "small", "good", "wrong", "something", "someone", "body", "you", "I", "people", "mine", "kind", "can", "maybe", "if", "inside", "live", and "die". Just as these words are common to all languages, so are the human experiences collected in the narration of stories of illness, daily life, and care [7].

Below the results collected by Alessandra Cecconello and Angela Micheli are shown:

> A total of 41 people took part in the project, including 16 young people, 6 parents, 13 teachers and 6 educators. The most represented average age of adolescents is between 14 and 17; for educators, it is 25; for parents and teachers, it is between 50 and 60. It emerged from all the narratives that the pandemic was, and still is, an individual and collective trauma that has left deep and yet unresolved traces in many individuals because it has caused a fracture in biographical linearity.
>
> Narrative medicine has allowed everyone to give voice to thoughts and states of mind that would otherwise have found no other possibility of expression. In essence, it has opened a window on experiences that are not investigated in other ways, which do not possess adequate tools to express themselves and, above all, ears interested in listening to them. The texts, for the most part, are constructed in descriptive, simple, and essential language. However, some children demonstrate a great capacity for reflection and introspection using more articulate and expressive language. The narratives have all been handwritten with distinctive styles (e.g., minute hand-

writing or broad and slender, organized in paragraphs extended to cover all available space or concentrated in one and a half lines). Corrections, exclamation marks, parentheses. Thoughts, observations, desires, dreams, certainties, an iridescent and lively world.

"Before Covid, it was very good, and I was freer; you could do more things outdoors. Then everything changed, and I felt caged. I could not have as much fun as before..."

"I miss going out with friends and spending time with them or visiting my grandmother."

"Now at school...come on, much better than before, even though sometimes it is boring. It is easier because if I need someone, there is someone who can help me, or I can study in peace. I like going out with friends downtown, hugging everyone, going on holiday; it is summer, so we go to the pool/sea."

And what did they tell us? Their well-being comes from creating and cultivating relationships, from physically "being" with their friends to following their interests and practicing their passions. These adolescents want and need to experience relationships physically, to have freedom of movement to expend the physical and intellectual energy typical of the age, which has curiosity, passions to follow and cultivate, and dreams to fulfil.

"I was happy before Covid because I had started my first year of high school. I could do many things, even though I could now take back what had been taken away from me. Staying at home, I felt bored, especially after a month, because this new lifestyle we all had to deal with through lockdown went from novelty to habit to boredom...

Now, I can see my classmates at school and no longer be half in front of a screen. At least now, lessons are easier to follow, and I can spend fewer hours behind screens. Studying is useful and indispensable to growing and maturing in one's life choices.

It makes me feel good to be with real people who do not make me feel lonely, to follow my passions and be myself 100% without filters, but above all, to dream and chase my dreams.

About school and studying, the difficulty perceived by adolescents with Distance Learning is unanimous. And not so much, or not only because of the medium itself but because of what it takes away from normal didactics: the closeness. The relationship, being physically together, and even studying. The most common adjectives used to describe studying were "difficult," "complicated," "tedious," and "tiring," often with the addition of "more."

Studying (Distance learning) was:

"Much more difficult than when we were at school".

"Tiring, tiring and unnecessary".

"Difficult and tiring, and you could not concentrate as much, especially having two brothers doing Distance Learning at the same time..."

"Difficult because I did not have the teachers with me".

> *"Complicated, in online classes, you couldn't always understand what the professor was explaining, so you had to study on your own".*
>
> *"Impossible; I couldn't focus, and I didn't feel like it".*
>
> And now? Studying is different. The terms that recur most frequently are easy, challenging, simple, and useful. And often still with the plus in front.
>
> *Studying is*
>
> *"Back to being normal"*
>
> *"Much easier"*
>
> *"Tiring, especially for some subjects, but with the right method, I do it without too many problems"*
>
> *"Easier because if I need help, there is someone who can help me, or I can study in peace".*
>
> *"Improved compared to middle school, thanks to the quarantine, I learnt to study on my own without the need to ask for help".*
>
> Three of the sixteen narratives describe major personal hardship situations that the pandemic has triggered or worsened:"
>
> *I was empty, apathetic, tired. I was strange as if I had a soup of emotions inside; it was tough to recognize them individually, and this caused me much anxiety. I had a perpetual knot in my throat".*
>
> What is also striking about the children is their attention to the problems of the environment and the contemporary world in general (war, pandemics, climate change).
>
> *"For the future, I would like a peaceful world without racism, a (cleaner) world, and to try to become a doctor".*
>
> *"I don't see much future; with climate change, COVID and many other problems, I don't know where we will end up. I fear having children because I cannot assure them the future they deserve".*
>
> *"For the future, I would like a life full of adventures and being outdoors a lot. Playing many sports, gaining a lot of experience, having a stable family with an honest, dynamic job that can meet my needs".* These narratives settled down the natural order of expectations concerning age, with the young projected towards tomorrow to conquer despite the dissonant voices.
>
> Youth are willing to share what they have been living, not wishing to spend too much time in schoolwork groups but looking forward to living in the open air and meeting with friends. Their parents are still worried and experiencing fatigue, as there was what we could collect as trauma for their living with teenagers at home. Some parents recall that experience of living at home as a "hell," which is not over yet.

I want to highlight this "Chaos Narrative," according to Arthur Frank [8]: "*I don't see much future, with climate change, covid and many other problems I don't know where we will end up.*" This could belong to teenagers or youth who call themselves

5.1 The Violence of Social Pressure   57

"Doomers," and this is a very worrying term. According to the urban dictionary, a *doomer* is characterized by a hostile stance towards the world, manifested mainly by a withdrawal from society. Doomers resent boomers and are aware of the great tragedies of life. They experience a phenomenon called Weltschmerz, which can be translated as the world's grief, indicating the deep sadness and melancholy one feels because of the world's imperfections (climate change, economic crisis, overpopulation). Doomers refuse to abandon suffering and cynicism and deny that there is a way out of the cycle of unhappiness. They consider the culprit of their sorrow mostly the Baby Boomer generation who was grid for welfare money, overexploited the planet, and gave rise to the worst conflicts of the Anthropocene age.

5.1.2 To Eat or Not to Eat, This Is the Problem

The lockdown periods were also associated with the onset of eating disorders in many youths. One aspect contributing to the notion that eating disorders (mainly anorexia and bulimia, avoidant behavior, and compulsive eating) constitute a hidden burden is inherent to the disorders themselves, like other mental disorders and obesity, eating disorders are associated with considerable stigma and self-stigmatization, typically as trivial and self-inflicted disorders. This stigma may hinder help-seeking behavior and contribute to a lower visibility and general lack of awareness of these disorders in society.

Results have shown that the global incidence of eating disorders increased during the COVID-19 pandemic by 15.3% in 2020 compared to previous years. The relative risk of eating disorders increased steadily from March 2020 onwards, exceeding 15% by the end of the year. The increase occurred only in women and girls and was observed mainly in adolescents and for anorexia nervosa: they are harming themselves, in a vicious cycle hard to break.

Here are some excerpts from interviews with a girl who started to suffer from anorexia when the pandemic started (Name is fictitious).

> *Rose is slightly nervous to talk about this, but she wants to. She sits next to her mom in their suburban, in Michigan. Her long, brown hair hangs loose over a red athletic jacket.*
> **Rose:** Yeah. So, my name is Rose. I am 15 years old. I play volleyball. About six months ago, I was diagnosed with anorexia nervosa.
> *Immediately, after these few words, she is silenced by the commenter who wants to clarify her situation.*
> **Journalist:** This disease has sent her to the emergency room four times. And she has been admitted to three different hospitals. It began in March of 2020 when the lockdown started. Suddenly, a girl who had been this athletic, high-achieving eighth grader just felt lost.

> **Rose:** People are dying. Everyone is getting sick. You can't see your friends. It was hard because I felt like I had no control over anything except what I ate and how I exercised.
>
> *The journalist gives us more details, somehow generalizing the behavior of the anorexic world:*
>
> **Journalist:** So, she was like, I'm just going to eat healthy. I'm going to stay in shape. But as the shutdowns and isolation stretched into summer, fall, and winter, her focus on food and exercise became more intense. It started to consume her. She would make these elaborate meals. And she'd post pictures to Instagram but then give them to her sister and lie and say she'd already eaten. She would skip time with friends to fit in yet another run. And she wore baggy sweats to cover up the weight loss. By January, Rose just felt drained and exhausted all the time.
>
> **Rose:** I had, like, basically no emotions. I was just, like, numb. All I wanted to do was, like, lay in my bed. And I finally said I am struggling with food. It was probably the hardest thing I've ever said in my entire life because I was so scared.
>
> **Journalist:** Rose was so sick 2 months later she needed to be admitted to the hospital. Hospitals across the country have seen a surge of patients like Rose.
>
> **Rose:** Being able to talk to people going through the same thing helped me realize that I am not alone. And I can - I'm starting to get activity back. I'm - I can hang out with my friends and live how I want. And I know it is tough to just, like, reach out. But at the end of the day, it's so worth it.
>
> The reading of the whole interview is moving because almost the entire room's attention was given to Rose. However, too many interruptions by the journalist are bringing bias to the narrative inquiry, which requires pure listening. In this interview, Rose is almost silenced by the journalist, please consider the length of each specific answer, the number of words; there is a didactic-didascalic chronicle of what "recipes" (nicknames for people suffering from anorexia) do or do not do.

Personally, I wish to find other ways to communicate with teenagers and young people. The generation gap feels enormous, and their expectations differ from those of Baby Boomers, Generation X, and Generation Y.

How do we help to get out of this anorexic-cycle of self-harm and construct a culture of non-invasive communication?

Exploring narrative medicine with girls battling anorexia, Dr. Merav Shohet, in Boston, is a Cultural Anthropologist specializing in Psychological, Medical, and Linguistic Anthropology [9]. She has been working in different contexts, such as the elderly and other marginalized social situations. She is a proponent of active

5.1 The Violence of Social Pressure

listening and empathizes with those suffering from anorexia. Exploring the narrative processes through which girls treated for anorexia reformulate their experiences of illness and recovery, the narratives are categorized into two distinct genres: "Full recovery" and "Struggling Recovery".

The analysis suggests that *full recovery* may involve a temporal disjunction between past and present selves and constructing a coherent empowerment narrative with clear beginnings, turning points, and happy, institutionally condoned endings.

Alternatively, the habitual narrative of equivocal narratives *struggling to recover*, in which protagonists question received wisdom, reflect on past and hypothetical life paths, and imagine starvation as both "good" and "bad," potentially perpetuating a cyclical life course in which anorexia repeats itself and permanent recovery eludes the narrators. Illuminating why complete recovery may remain ephemeral and, perhaps, undesirable for some women, this article contributes to scholarship on storytelling's possible role (and limitations) as a therapeutic means and resource for coping with illness.

Here is how Dr. Shohet allows girls to speak: please note that the (.) means pause.

Interviewer: And at the time did you resent it...you know that she pulled it out and moved it and everything?
Violet (is a fictitious name): A bit. Well, a bit...
Because...I want – I was never sure I wanted to give up the eating disorder. But cause, at one point, all my life was (.) was the eating disorder. I knew nothing else and what I did know I didn't like, I didn't like where I was before, so...I was committing sub-conscious suicide basically...But in the back of my head, I knew...I was happy that they were helping me.
Umm, my personality, my behaviors always (.) focused on (.) ummm (.) being perfect, overachieving, very typical case scenario, and this because my family was having those dysfunctions.

The interview, based on anthropologic and soft skills, is prone to being a facilitator of the story of the involved people. Develops and Violet says:

> I always think that there are two things that I have that no one can take away from me, and (.) that's my choice- I can choose to do something, I can choose to eat something, I can choose not to eat something, I can choose to go out with someone, or not, and my voice- I can tell you how I feel, and I can tell myself.

The interviewer does not interrupt this free flow of consciousness, which reveals a great awareness in Violet. What is evident in the mind of the observer is that there is a clear cut between the past, with the wounds of willingness to overachieve in a dysfunctional family, and the present, which, starting from the food, includes the possibility of eating/not eating, overachieving or just achieving. Dr. Shohet brings another narrative, which is a story that she does not define as of recovery since there is no change, *"All my life, and still now, to like myself, I need good feedback... I don't know...If only I did not have the label"*, these are just a few words from a second "stuck story". As you can see, there is no discontinuation between the past and the present.

Now the Psychological centers are overwhelmed with young population with eating disorders, panic attacks, or *"decision to leave"* (this world)-attempts to suicide [10].

5.2 Invitation to Live

Hebe, the goddess of youth and spring in the phylogenesis of the myth, is the daughter of Zeus and his wife Hera. She does not belong to the old progenies but to the new ones. Hebe wants to flourish, to live in social banquets, and to entertain others with beauty and grace.

We should be worried since too many students in 2022 prefer distance learning, 8 out of 10 students to be specific (although the survey I am referring to is possibly biased since a distance learning university carried it out) (14). This is yet an alarming result because most of the social life is precluded, there are still so many new encounters and possibilities, at this age. Not to mention, the brain is still in development. The advantage is efficiency and lower cost, but this price does not include the poor health outcomes that counteract the benefits.

The invitation is to get out of this society at risk of Hikikomori since the results of distance learning are right before our eyes. More than 500,000 young Italian people quit academic study in the last 3 years! If it is true that the pandemic was a catalyzer of our digitalization skills, the very self-digitalization should not become our trap. Despite the impressive capabilities of today's "web village," with a face for a zoom gaze, we do have a real physical body; we have an environment around us, neighbors, trains, low carbon emission planes to catch, and the beauty of the world to see. The apparent agoraphobia is syndemic with the virus infection. The first pandemic is over, we have to learn to find a sustainable balance between real-life interaction and distance learning, "smart working," and other digital skills, which could be key generators to the observed trends of loneliness, anxiety, and depression, which are higher now than ever before.

How can older generations invite, in a nonviolent way, the youth to open themselves to live real-life experiences since too many are comfortable with 7 days a week of "smart working" without feeling the need for social interactions? We may focus on the burden of this social interaction and pressure on teenagers.

I will never be able to express in words and deeds enough gratitude to the young generation for their sacrifice of locking themselves down during the pandemic. They shielded themselves to save our generations and older generations; they were in the narrative study "Narrating vaccination," an excellent altruistic example since, to get their freedom, they wanted to be vaccinated by whatever means. Now they need our help, and no blaming culture, that labels them as "cold-hearted spoiled losers." Open the window to Emily Dickinson, with her entourage of Hikikomori and anorexia survivors/warriors, girls who spread themselves thin for the sake of others and let her spirit flow over the Hamster countryside. Let us imagine that she dares, to go downstairs barefoot, open the main door and get outside, to walk in that

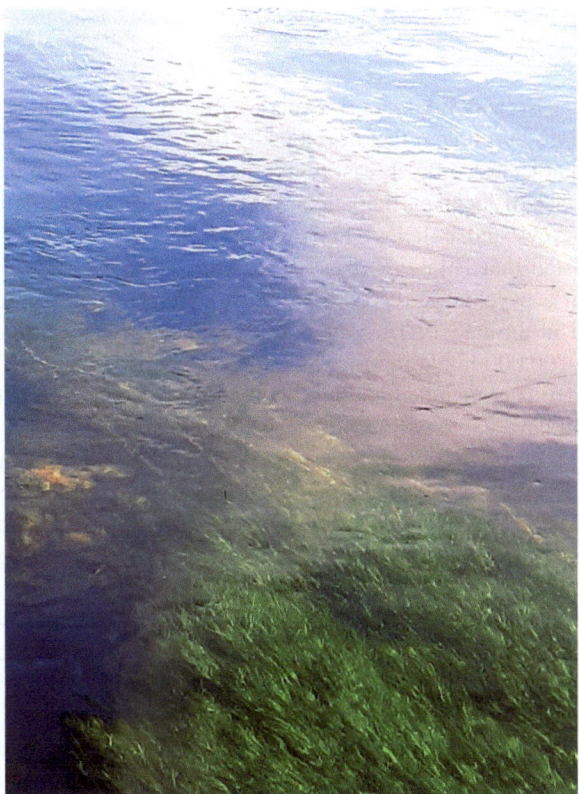

Fig. 5.1 River hair (photo by Maria Giulia Marini)

clover prairies, and listen to frogs speaking, and the bees go buzzing, with no funeral in her mind, with a clear view of yesterday, today and tomorrow (Fig. 5.1).

5.3 Practice Time

1.
> When K-san (52) wakes up in the morning, there is a note on the kitchen table from his younger son, T, who is 21 years old. The note reads, "I want a guitar string." In the middle of the night, Tomo sneak's downstairs to write notes because he cannot hold a real conversation with his parents. K-San, T's father, is a civil servant in Hokkaido. He, his wife (47), and his son live together. In the summer of his first year of high school, Tomo dropped out, and soon after, he shut himself away in his room. "We have not had a meal together once in the past four years," his father says. Tomo hides in his room and avoids showing his face. He carries his food to his room, locks the door behind him, and eats there. He has been afraid of meeting people for the past four years and does not go outside. He spends every night plucking at his guitar. At the end of last year, Tomo expressed the wish to go outside.

It seemed as though he wanted to rejoin society. But this, too, he communicated in a note.—
S Y (1997)

The psychiatrist and hikikomori expert Saito Tamaki's initial definition of Hikikomori as "a problem that develops by the time an individual is in his late twenties (characterized by at least 6 months of withdrawal into the home and a continuing lack of social participation" [11]) laid the groundwork for future government surveys and policies [12]. Although he is a psychiatrist, Saitoˆ has always insisted that Hikikomori is a condition (joˆtai), a state of being, not a symptom of a psychiatric disorder [13]. He estimated there were one million Hikikomori in the late 1990s, although a Cabinet survey in 2010 revised that estimate to 700,000 hikikomori among youth between the ages of 15 and 34, a number that did not include 'potential' Hikikomori who are averse to social relationships but have yet to withdraw completely.

At a Hikikomori Discussion Group (HDG), where the only given assignment was "free talk", neither parents nor Hikikomori ever claimed the hikikomori experience itself was pleasant, but there were parents in the HDG who read into Hikikomori a significance that *transformed it from social failure to profound psychological experience*. One night, during the group's post-meeting gathering at a local fast-food restaurant, a middle-aged male hikikomori became drunk and raucous. He burped loudly, insisted he was still sober, and proclaimed he had a 15-year-old boy's psychological age (Seishin nenrei). The group leader, a mother in her early sixties whose grey hair was dyed with a dusting of rose blush, protested. "Hikikomori," she said, "have a higher psychological age than their peers because they spend so much time thinking about life."

Framed in this light, the Hikikomori display a wisdom beyond their years, performing the difficult psychological work of self-discovery that takes others a lifetime to achieve. Sometimes, the hikikomori period acquired the mystical qualities of a religious experience. A 60-year-old mother whose 29-year-old son had been a hikikomori in his third year of junior high school narrated that Hikikomori emerged after their withdrawal period. Now plotted as a psychological journey, Hikikomori is not simply a passive reaction to a pathological society but can potentially be a volitional act of self-discovery. However, not all parents can understand Hikikomori or maintain a sense of narrative time, especially when the Hikikomori period dragged on for years or decades without any signs of change.

(a) Which of these lines above inspired you? Think about a possible withdrawal experience from a society of one of your patients, one of your family members, or yourself. Now apply reflective writing: 20 lines, to say what happened, the deeds, the words, the untold, the location, the emotions, the symbols, the projects…in particular, reflect upon Hikikomori as a possible reaction to "the violence" of society, bullies, narcissist, verbal or physical abuse. Could Hikikomori be a consequence of trauma?

5.3 Practice Time

(b) Now, think of a nonviolent communication (NVC) dialogue with a person who lives with Hikikomori, but more than living it as a contemplation process, in essence, lives it as an addiction to nocturnal video games. Please refer to the four domains of the biological, psychological, social and existential model. The four steps are a reality check, an analysis of the emotions, needs, and expression of requests by both sides.

A Japanese survey 2022 revealed that approximately 1.46 million people, or 2% of the Japanese population between 15 and 64, could be living as *Hikikomori* (i.e. modern-day hermits) in the country. The large number of social recluses is considered a significant social issue in Japan, and the growing number of *Hikikomori* has raised concerns in government and the private sector, especially as the country's labor force continues to shrink. So thinking to our contemporary society the Hikikomori condition is pervasive and crosses the generations, arriving to our "smart worker" generations.

2. Students of your acquaintance want to quit their studies, for different reasons, some because there are bothered by studying, some because they want to find a job, and some because they don't want to do anything. Or maybe other reasons.

I, myself...
I feel...
Now I want...
My people...
At school/ university...
In my free time...
For the future I want...
Think about their parents; what about collecting their narratives using these prompts? (Please use one plot for every child of this family.)
I, myself...
I feel...
I want
My child...
He/she feels...
He/she wants...
My people...
His/her people..
At school/university...
In my free time...
In his/her free time
For the future I want...
For the future he/she wants...

Read if inside the stories there is rage and/or low self-esteem. What kind of emotions might lead to self-harm and violence towards others? Discover while reading also all the inner resources, the hobbies, the interests, wishes, the people they love and channel their Stories towards these constructive and not destructive energy.

If you are the health care professional of young people and you are facing difficulties in establishing a connection with the young generation, what kind of communication style would you establish with them?

References

1. James O. Juvenile violence in a winner-loser culture: socio-economic and familial origins of the rise in violence against the person. London Free Association Book; 1995.
2. Wu S, Zhang K, Parks-Stamm EJ, Hu Z, Ji Y, Cui X. Increases in anxiety and depression during COVID-19: a large longitudinal study from China. Front Psychol. 2021;
3. Dong X-X, Li D-L, Miao Y-F, Zhang T, Yibo W, Pan C-W. The COVID-19 outbreak, with a depression prevalence of 43.7% among Chinese adolescents. J Affect Disord. 2023;333:1–9.
4. Caso D, Guidetti M, Capasso M, Cavazza N. Finally, the chance to eat healthily: longitudinal study about food consumption during and after the first COVID-19 lockdown in Italy. Food Qual Prefer. 2021;
5. Marini MG. The languages of care in narrative medicine. Acura di Springer; 2019.
6. Frank A. The wounded storyteller: body, illness and ethics. University Chicago Press; 1997.
7. Shohet M. Beyond the clinic? Eluding a medical diagnosis of anorexia through narrative. Transcult Psychiatry. 2018;55(4):495–515.
8. https://www.nationwidechildrens.org/newsroom/newsreleases/2023/02/bridge_ruch_youthsuicide
9. Masalimova AR, Khvatova MA, Chikileva LS, Zvyagintseva EP, Stepanova VV, Melnik MV. Distance learning in higher education during Covid-19. Front Educ. 2022;
10. Tamaki, Saito. n.d.. https://en.wikipedia.org/wiki/Hikikomori#:~:text=The%20psychiatrist%20Tamaki%20Sait%C5%8D%20defines%20hikikomori%20as%20%22a,have%20another%20psychological%20problem%20as%20its%20principal%20source%22.
11. Ellen Rubbstein, Emplotting Hikikomori: Japanese parents' narratives of social withdrawal, culture, medicine and psychiatry; 2016.
12. Teo AR. A new form of social withdrawal in Japan: a review of Hikikomori. Int J Soc Psychiatry. 2016;
13. https://www.researchgate.net/publication/314285140_Hikikomori_The_Japanese_Cabinet_Office's_2016_Survey_of_Acute_Social_Withdrawal

Chapter 6
Nonviolent Communication with the Older People, Honoring Them During Their Last Years, and The Violence of Agism

In Greek mythology, Geras (hence, we derive the words "geriatrics" and "gerontology" from ancient Greek) was the god of old age. He was depicted as a tiny, shriveled old man. Gēras' opposite was Hebe, a beautiful girl, the goddess of youth. Hebe served nectar and ambrosia to all gods and goddesses on Mount Olympus. On the contrary, Geras did not serve anything sweet, rather he served the fear of becoming frail, old, and dying. His Roman equivalent was Senectus (thus, we derive words such as "Senior" and "Senatus"). For the Greeks, Geras was also a metaphor for disability, he is often depicted while leaning on a cane. However, from the pragmatic Latin viewpoint, being old gave access to wisdom, and therefore, political power in the Senatum. A "Senior," then, became a person who deserves respect, and "Seniority," a quality to appreciate. The status symbol of being old is acknowledged by the Latin word "antianus" which means *more history*: form here the word "ancient," "ancienne," and in Italian "anziano."

For the English word, "old" comes from *ald* (Anglian), *eald* (West Saxon, Kentish) "antique, of ancient origin, belonging to antiquity, primeval; long in existence or use; near the end of the normal span of life; elder, mature, experienced," from Proto-Germanic **althaz* "grown up, adult."

Evaluating the ancestor's trees of gods and goddess, Geras was born from Nox (Night) and Erebus, the personification of darkness and shadow. Some of their brothers and sisters were Fatum (Fate), Thanatos (Death)—we have met him in his dedicated chapter—Hypnos (Sleep), Oneiroi (Dreams), Amor (Love), Discordia / Eris (Discord), Hybris (Wantonness), Gratia, Nemesis (Envy), Euphrosyne (Good Cheer), Philotes (Friendship), Eleos (Compassion), Styx (Hate); the three Parcae (Fates), and the Hesperides.

This complexity of brotherhood and sisterhood, of human qualities, and events is simply breathtaking. From the same parents, the offspring can represent getting old as being lovely and compassionate or conflictual and hateful.

© The Author(s), under exclusive license to Springer Nature
Switzerland AG 2024
M. G. Marini, *Non-violent Communication and Narrative Medicine for Promoting Sustainable Health*, New Paradigms in Healthcare,
https://doi.org/10.1007/978-3-031-58691-0_6

Geras is not considered only as a source of frailty, but as embodied in humans, represented a virtue: the more *gēras* (old) a man acquired, the more *kleos* (fame) and *arete* (excellence and courage) he was considered to have. In ancient Greek literature, the related word *géras* can also mean influence, authority or power, mainly that derived from fame, good looks, and strength claimed through success in battle or contest. Such uses of this meaning can be found in Homer's *Odyssey*, throughout which there is an evident concern from the various kings about the *géras* they will pass to their sons through their names.

The problem is significant because kings, at this time (such as Odysseus), were believed to have ruled by common consent in recognition of their powerful influence rather than hereditarily.

When we go through this philological analysis, we learn that the culture that gave more meaning to this word to the elderly is Greek. Aging could have been a status of wisdom, a realm of confusion, fear, and darkness, and facing liminality.

6.1 The Threshold of Elderly Today

What criteria is used to define an "old person"? The United Nations defines "older persons" as those aged 60 years or over. On many occasions, it is defined as 65+: "Age 65 is generally set as the threshold of old age since it is at this period of life that the rates for sickness and death begin to show a marked increase in comparison to those of earlier years" [1].

Suppose a man living in Western Europe is going to celebrate his 60th birthday, is he old? Today, this person would be considered middle-aged, and around 93% of men survive until that age. About 150 years ago, less than 25% (of men, of the general population, were celebrating their 60th birthday. Indeed, at those times, someone at age 60 was considered an old man. The traditional age measure is a backward-looking one. It tells us how many years a person has already lived. However, this is an incomplete measure because it ignores changes in life expectancy. "Young" and "old" are relative notions; their standard reference point is life expectancy. Using the concept of perspective age, we can state that someone who is 60 today may be equivalent to someone who was 43 years old in 1850. A person who was 60 years old 150 years ago may resemble someone who is 74 today.

Essentially, we recognized people as having two different ages: a chronological age, defined also as a "retrospective age," which measures how many years a person has lived. Everyone in the same period has lived the same number of years. In contrast, "prospective age" is concerned with the future. Everyone with the same prospective age has the same expected remaining years. Population ageing will undoubtedly be the source of many challenges in the twenty-first century. Every year lived, or expected to live, is not only quantitative, but also qualitative. If life expectancy before COVID-19 was continuously increasing up until 2019, it is interesting to assess the way "old people" lived these past years. Some studies show that although life is prolonged, the quality of the last years might be poor. Public and private investment in medical research is primarily focused on reducing death rates rather than reducing ageing and age-related diseases. As Guy Brown writes in "Living too long":

> *Even in the absence of disease and disability, human abilities—including memory, cognition, mobility, sight, hearing, taste and communication—decline with age), so the quality of life for someone older than 90 years is very poor. Given the increasing prevalence of multiple diseases, disabilities, dementias and dysfunctions at high age, it is not obvious that just extending lifespan beyond 90 years of age is worthwhile* [2].

I know maybe we might be shocked reading the lines above, and the more I go through this topic, the more I think about what narrative medicine is for: to escape the confinement of a standardized biomedical model, and instead, incorporate the biological, social, psychological, and existential dimensions of multifaced and multipage period life to the practice of medicine.

6.2 The Witnessing of Living with Elders with Alzheimer

Worldwide, Alzheimer's and Dementia affects around 40 million people, and in Italy, there are about one million cases, mostly over 60 years of age. Over the age of 80, one in four elderly people is affected [3]. These digits will eventually increase, given the ageing of the population.

In the REMIND [4] action learning project by ISTUD in 2022, 16 neurology clinicians from centers of excellence in Italy in treating Alzheimer's disease were engaged in collaborative research studying and applying narrative medicine.

The narrative illness plots were co-constructed with the class to collect three points of view, that of people living with Alzheimer's, their caregivers and their doctors.

The physicians collected 43 narratives: 12 from patients, 12 from relatives, and 18 parallel charts by doctors. From the analysis, it emerged that patients, especially when diagnosed early, can narrate their living with Alzheimer's in writing, indicating their primary fear, which is the loss of memories, especially affective memories. They are moderately unaware of the burden of care given to their "caregivers" and often turn to their own intimate, world, even with those closest to them. It appears they are in "another world," making it tough to be accepted and understood by their proxies. In their narrative the most present word is "NOT" which means a function to make negative the possibility to speak, to act, but Not to think they are aware of the fact that *"they cannot,"* and exceptionally, using the simple universal words of the NSM, they were able to put it into writing. They need contact; *"I would like to hug"; and* they feel a nostalgic sentiment *"To be able to go back."*

Despite their few words, this awareness of their condition, which eventually will deteriorate, and therefore, calls for help from people around them.

The caregivers, the fragile link in the system, write of the fatigue and weariness of staying "so long" next to the person they "no longer recognize," and who "no longer recognizes them," feeling highjacked. It was found that anger was the dominant emotion expressed in response to this "unfair" change, sadness and compassion followed. Examples of responses conveying anger were, *"Our relationship is very conflictual,"* and *"the situation at times has led to misunderstandings and difficult moments."* Caregivers confessed that their anger was mainly due to the "different" behavior of their loved one: *'his mind is a mystery. I am convinced there is a swarm of other "faces" of her in there that I have never seen.'* If we consider the wish for contact by persons with Alzheimer's from their narratives, we might find a misalignment with the caregiver's astonishment.

Both patients and caregivers fear the "unexpected" and the possible "shaming" by their other relatives and broader society: *"She only wants to go to protected spaces, where she knows people. At lunch, she wants to know who is there, and if there are strangers, she doesn't come... she who was full of friends and so active in volunteering. Her perimeter has shrunk,"* *"People who once were close to us have gone away."*

The services that only partially care for the needs of a person with Alzheimer's are another cause for anger because it creates additional unnecessary responsibilities for the family. In this way, family members risk not only losing their loved one, but also, sacrificing much of their own life: *"And alone, powerless against something that overpowered me and demolished every certainty I had had up to that point. The doctors told us that there was no chance of recovery and that the only hope of slowing down the disease came from experimental protocols."* *"I live day by day; I prefer not to think of any tomorrow."*

Vulnerability was a reoccurring theme that emerged in the narratives of physicians, contrary to what one might think of their status and role. In fact, they revealed that they often felt "disarmed" since there are currently no known treatments that work effectively against Alzheimer's: *"the feeling I generally feel when I communicate the diagnosis is one of unease (although I never give it away), linked to the inexorability of the diagnosis."* Yet, as the reflection on the narratives proceeded, the potential of a new way of being a doctor emerged, namely caring for not only for life but for patients' existence, whatever it may be. Not only of the person with Alzheimer's disease but also of his/her family member: *"You get sick in two, love can be very painful;"* *"I always get close. I think you can't stay distant even with your body. I always look for 'closeness.'"* Accompanying, pushing for association, teaching, and managing emotions, mourning the loss of identities for the reconstruction of new identities, no longer delegated to psychologists but also dealt with in neurology practices: *"I hope in the future I can continue to be a comfort and help to them."*

According to the mentioned report "Living too long," there should be no room for these old people with lost identity (possibly from the narratives of another one) in a cruel society in which close people and friends abandon the "Alzheimer's pair," and both confines themselves in a very tiny perimeter. However, there is so much need for intelligent love, for caregivers who do not demand, nor expect to receive the persons they had once in their life; those who are not ashamed of "the oddities" that people with Alzheimer's express in public. Equally as important is the need for intelligent care by doctors who are not worried by the fact that there is no medication, who acknowledge the different identities of the patients, and refrain from speaking only about "loss." And yes, there is possibility to live longer, in whatever condition.

6.3 The Isolation Damages

Until Covid-19, ageing was challenging but not so fearful and risky. The virus is especially lethal for the elderly: "Average American life expectancy dropped precipitously in 2020 and 2021. In 2021, the average American could expect to live to the age of 76…a loss of almost three years from 2019, when Americans could expect to live, on average, almost 79 years. The reduction was particularly sharp among Native Americans and Alaska Natives, the National Centre for Health Statistics reported. Average life expectancy in these groups dropped by four years in 2020 alone. The cumulative decline since the start of the pandemic, averaging more than six and a half years, has brought life expectancy to 65 years among Native Americans and Alaska Natives, on par with that of all Americans in 1944." Possibly, this was mainly due to the poor access to vaccination of people excluded by public health programs.

While in 2020 compared to 2019, average life expectancy, for both men and women, in Italy had fallen from 83.6 years to 82.3 years. In 2021, provisional data indicated a recovery with life expectancy rising to 82.9 years. The most significant decreases were estimated in Slovakia and Bulgaria (−2.2 years compared to 2020), followed by Latvia (−2.1) and Estonia (−2.0). However, compared to the pre-pandemic year of 2019, the overall effect is still negative in all Member States except Luxembourg, Malta and Sweden.

It was a nightmare, and during that age, the main messages given to the elderly people to survive were: "shield yourself," a euphemism that meant, "don't see anybody," using the too obvious metaphoric battle language (take a shield).

A research team of UCL [5] used data from more than 5000 adults aged over 50 who are part of the English Longitudinal Study of Ageing (ELSA) to investigate the link between shielding and mental health after controlling for sociodemographic characteristics, pre-pandemic physical and psychological health, and social isolation measures. The data was collected during the first 8–9 months of the pandemic, two of which were characterized by ongoing lockdowns. Respondents were asked whether in April, June/July, and November/December 2020 they shielded (not going out of the house for any reason), stayed at home (leaving only for minimal purposes, such as shopping for food, exercise, or essential work) or neither. Their mental health was then assessed by asking about depressive symptoms, anxiety, well-being, and quality of life.

About 28% of respondents reported shielding at least once, with 5% shielding throughout the first 8/9 months of the pandemic. About a third reported staying at home all the time, whereas 37% neither shielded nor stayed at home. Among those adults who always covered, in November and December 2020, 42% reported elevated depressive symptoms compared to 23% who never shielded nor stayed at home. Older people shielded throughout the period studied also reported the lowest life satisfaction and quality of life scores.

The researchers were able to account for pre-pandemic mental and physical health as well as for social contacts with family and friends and loneliness during the pandemic to better understand if the relationships observed between shielding and poorer mental health were driven by pre-existing conditions or reduced social interactions and higher loneliness during the pandemic.

Of course, on the one hand, there is depression; on the other, there is the risk of COVID-19 death, but that depression also caused many cardiovascular accidents and neurodegenerative diseases as dementia, diminishing the chance of maintaining the opportunity of well-being in this already vulnerable group.

And this connects with our basic needs, the social interconnection to flourish, live, and survive.

6.3.1 Agism, A Short-Sighted Prejudice

I met many years ago, in 1999, Rita Levi Montalcini, the Italian Nobel Prize for Medicine on Nervous Growth Factor. She was *only ninety* years old; she died at 103 years. She was asked to give a lecture, and walking through the congress hall with a cane, gave no PowerPoint presentation, but a "stream of consciousness" speech for thirty minutes. Everyone was fascinated by her charisma and her inspirational words devoted to research and healthcare professionals. She never lost herself in the address; she was stunning. One could argue that she had the tools; she was a Nobel prize. True; however, I think that what she did is that she accepted, without shame, the fact that she walked with a cane, that she wore a hearing aid and glasses—the signs of "body aging." Her soul and mind were so great, she was living proof of the reasons why she won the prize, a prime example of neuroplasticity. Is it easy to come to this age like Prof. Montalcini? Not at all. It required discipline in lifestyle, from the food we eat to our selfcare practices, and the hard intellectual work we choose to engage in every day.

These lines are devoted to all elderly people who, despite their bodies falling to pieces, as Lucien Freud painted in his portraits, are practicing every day, doing soft gym, crosswords, helping with grandchildren and great-grandchildren, writing, lecturing, cooking, cleaning...their narratives are essential and witnessing the wish to leave a legacy, when the last years are fading away.

Rita Levi Montalcini left everything to research neuroplasticity. Again, the prejudice of becoming greedy with age is only a wrong judgement and not a proper evaluation.

6.4 Narrative Medicine with Elderly in Nursing Home

Narratives of old people are often looking backwards to the past, in a Proustian style, "searching the lost time," or Miltonian "searching the lost paradise." They exude nostalgia from almost every word. When we collect the narratives, we set four basic prompts: *"Before I was…" "It happened that…," "Now…"and, "For the future"…*, using the NSM words in a diachronic mode. Of course, they are adapted to the circumstances in which elderly people find themselves. However, in different contexts, their narratives often have a very constrained "Now" and a lacking future.

Here are some narratives from a nursing home in Northern Italy collected by an occupational therapist:

Woman, 95 years old

> *I can tell you that my life has been good, good, well-defined. I worked, I got married when I was 19, and I went into a shop and came out after 40 years. I had a bakery, my husband baked with the workers, and I sold the products to the shop assistant. I had five or six workers, and I worked a lot. It was nice, beautiful. I worked a lot, but I never felt tired; there was enthusiasm. I am enthusiastic about my life…In the future, what do you want me to see? I'm 95 years old, I'm happy with everything, I read crosswords, and I'm fine. It's just long to get through the days. Then there's my daughter, who helps me so much. I have everything I need, and she doesn't let me lack anything.*

Here is a woman who lived a good life; she is just how "bothered" by the day-by-day routine. Possibly, there is a huge amount untold in this narrative…what would she like to do during the days? And would she like to go on, enduring this boredom? She clearly says, "In my future, what do you want me to see?" Nonetheless, she talks about the future carried on by the wonderful, dedicated daughters. This is one of the ways in which elderly people speak about the future: mentioning future generations.

Man, 84 years old

> *For 15 years as a plumber, I worked among people and liked it. Then when I went to people's homes, I understood whether they could pay or not. We had a different mentality. If I saw that they had a nice house, I would make the right price; if they couldn't, I would ask for the labor to make a living, not to make money. I asked very little. When there was a flood, I changed all the installations for those who needed it. I would put it on the burner and not charge for the work. They came to ring my bell because I was honest.*

In this narrative there is no gazing at the future: the past was the land of values and honesty; the price of the reparation would have been tailored to the availability of money for paying.

A nonviolent communication strategy would collect this narrative by using these open prompts:

Tell me about yourself, about your life before arriving here.
How did you come to this facility (the nursing home)?
How did you feel in the beginning?
Tell me about you now, about your life here.
What would you like for tomorrow?

The four steps of Nonviolent communication are all here: the acknowledgement of the facts, emotions, needs, and, therefore, the possibility of compromise on the needs. Maybe, asking the biography before the nursing home, the feeling for the arrival in a "last place of life," the asking about how life is there... and the thoughts about tomorrow could help the guests in this social and clinical setting. Here are the words of what the occupational therapist learned by using the prompts listed above:

> Each narrative has given me back so much. It helped me discover sides I did not know about the people involved. For example, with the former plumber, with moments of severe psychomotor agitation, I met an old friend of hers who lives a few steps away from the facility, and we occasionally visit her for a chat and coffee. On the way back, he is quieter and for a few days, if you stick to the meeting, it is easier to manage daily. ...Instead, with one lady, I learned about her sadness, completely changing my idea about her before I knew her narration.
>
> The moment of narration was not just an educational and informative moment for me but also a pleasant episode for the facility's residents: they felt important because someone was interested in their lives, their emotions, their thoughts, and their outbursts.

Making the people worth telling to be listened could be a main activity of the social and health care workers in these facilities: in this way, the memories of their lives on this planet will not get lost. The "guests" in this nursing home did not win any Nobel prizes; they were plumbers, bakers, and rice harvesters. They came from a very poor and humble region. However, thanks to the "stubbornness" of some members of the equipe who wanted to introduce narrative competence as listening, recording, asking, being curious, and being respectful of their past, they managed to improve the guests' present. People who never wanted to play cards with the others were, after the narrative experience, involved in much more social life within the facility. Overall, this nursing home had a more relaxed atmosphere and became a center for specially tailored projects. As for the plumber, he went to go visit an old friend off-site., together with the social worker, accomplishing his need.

6.5 The Natural Threshold

Is the natural ecosystem all 'good'? Not at all, violence is made of the alternation of life and death, the abandonment of premature animals, and catastrophes that eradicate all forms of life, with ageing with the body falling apart. Giacomo Leopardi writes well about it, calling nature a stepmother [6].

O nature, nature
Why do you not then render?
What do you promise then?

Nature took Silvia—his beloved-away at too young, a flower that blossomed and fell before Summer.

Generally, the alternation of the cycle of the seasons offers nature growth, full of AUXINS and Chlorophyll (the substances that make plants lush and green), then transmutation, with the Xanthophylls of autumn coloring the leaves from green to yellow until the loss of winter, symbolically identified as an old man in ancient culture who must then meet his end. In some traditions, *he* is beheaded—to make room for the new generation of girls representing spring. And so, in cycles.

Those terrible limits that Leopardi saw in 'stepmotherly nature' can be reconfigured into other philosophies that are more conciliatory, compassionate, and helpful in healing. Let us consider the limit imposed by death as a neutral condition without giving it such a negative meaning. Our society is sometimes too unrealistic (not aware of the laws of nature) and too ideologized and mythomaniacal (Prometheus unchained, unleashed and not "chained"), with access to all technological possibilities, until it will be Artificial Intelligence—whose first ancestor was the discovery of fire given by Prometheus, a discovery that would no longer render Sapiens as useless, but immortal.

We know the World Health Organization's declaration defines well-being as a complete state of psycho-physical and social well-being: well, let us agree on how many years of longevity we mortal beings are "entitled" to. Suppose we want to counter the ineluctable ageing of the mind and body. How can we accept the limitation without making ourselves potentially infantile and mad with the desire to take the place of the gods?

From Eastern philosophies and religions, we learn that funeral rites in Tibet and Nepal are performed by feeding the corpse to vultures, "the scavengers," or by burning it and scattering the ashes on the fields as fertilizer to nourish the earth. The ashes in the wind symbolize the beauty of impermanence, the medicine against the boredom of eternity. We read it in the wise narratives of the seriously ill or in the very old who feel that the stalk of their leaf is about to fall off. They prepare themselves for the blowing of the wind, not wishing to be over-medicated; they want to be left in peace, no longer having to prove themselves by undergoing yet another treatment (acting in opposition of the Progeny of Prometheus Unleashed-Unchained).

I'm grateful to Prometheus because, thanks to him, we have learnt to warm ourselves at night, stop panicking in the cold, and cook (Levi Strauss' demarcation between raw and cooked). Of course, he saw ahead, but we Sapiens were not so strategic and ethical in using everything that comes and goes from Progress, nor in respecting the laws of Nature, Life and Death.

6.6 Practice Time

1. Violent narratives in nursing homes are events which happen. Seven kinds of abuse mainly occur [7]

   - Abandonment
   - Emotional abuse
   - Financial exploitation

- Neglect of a resident's basic needs
- Physical abuse
- Self-neglect
- Sexual assault

The sadness of these events is that it is very difficult to encourage the residents to speak boldly, as they find themselves in a constant condition of vulnerability and fragility. They must protect themselves from the violence of verbal abuse and even the possibility of blackmail—if they speak out they may lose their right to be adequately washed, dressed, nourished, and undressed. This causes traumas in elderly people, and this was an existing issue before the deadly pandemic. It is reported that the current health crisis has particularly affected the elderly population: Nursing homes have unfortunately experienced a relatively large number of deaths during the COVID-19 pandemic [7]. Based on this observation and work, we wanted to check whether nursing homes lent themselves to excess mortality even before the pandemic. Controlling for many essential characteristics of the elderly population in and outside nursing homes, we conjecture that the difference in mortality between those two samples was attributed to how nursing homes are designed and organized. Using matching methods, excess mortality was reported in Sweden, Belgium, Germany, Switzerland, Czech Republic, and Estonia, but not in the Netherlands, Denmark, Austria, France, Italy and Spain. This raises the question of the organization and management of these nursing homes and their design and financing. We know the pandemic severely hit Italy and Spain, and many residents died in 2020; however, we could speculate that a "human touch" to the care administered in these nursing homes would have reduced incident rate for any one of the seven abuses taking place in these three Mediterranean countries.

What would you like to change to improve the quality of care to the elderly in nursing homes through Humanities for Health and Nonviolent Communication Skills?

2. Sailing to Byzantium
    William Butler Yeats
    That is no country for old men. The young
    In one another's arms, birds in the trees,
    —Those dying generations—at their song,
    The salmon falls, the mackerel-crowded seas,
    Fish, flesh, or fowl, commend all summer long
    Whatever is begotten, born, and dies.
    Caught in that sensual music, all neglect
    Monuments of unageing intellect.
    II
    An aged man is but a paltry thing,
    A tattered coat upon a stick unless
    Soul clap its hands and sing, and louder sing
    For every tatter in its mortal dress,

Nor is there a singing school, but studying
Monuments of its own magnificence;
And therefore, I have sailed the seas and come
To the holy city of Byzantium.
III
sages standing in God's holy fire
As in the gold mosaic of a wall,
Come from the holy fire, perne in a gyre,
And be the singing masters of my soul.
Consume my heart away; sick with desire
And fastened to a dying animal
It knows not what it is; and gathers me
Into the artifice of eternity.
IV
Once out of nature, I shall never take
My bodily form from any natural thing,
But such a form as Grecian goldsmiths make
Of hammered gold and gold enamelling
To keep a drowsy Emperor awake;
Or set upon a golden bough to sing
To lords and ladies of Byzantium
Of what is past, or passing, or to come.

This is a poem by the Irish poet Yeats. As a side note: Don't worry for the English, which might be pretty tricky to understand. Search for this poem in Google, and with DEEPL, you can translate it into your language.

What does this poem inspire in you? Do you think that it could help cope with ageing?

3. Agism

Jonathan Swift describes in The Gulliver's Travels, in the lines of "Living too long" in Chap. 26, the *struldbrugg*—those humans in the nation of Luggnagg who are born seemingly normal but are immortal. Although *struldbruggs* do not die, they do continue ageing. Upon reaching the age of eighty (parametrized to the XVIII century life expectancy), they become legally dead and suffer from many ailments, including the loss of eyesight and hair.

As soon as they have completed the term of eighty years, they are looked on as dead in law; their heirs immediately succeed to their estate. After that period, they are held incapable of any employment of trust or profit. They cannot purchase lands or take leases, neither are they allowed to be witnesses in any cause, either civil or criminal or economic, not even for the decision of metes and bounds.

This is ruled since Swift writes that avarice is the necessary consequence of old age, and those immortals, if not stopped, would in time become proprietors of the whole nation and engross the civil power, which, for want of abilities to manage, must end in the ruin of the public.

What do you think about this possible Swift's "ageism"? Could it be an objective evaluation and a prejudiced and stereotyped way of judging the elderly?

Would you like to listen, collect and interpret the narratives of old people among your patients, colleagues, relatives and friends?

References

1. https://www.un.org/en/development/desa/population/events/pdf/expert/29/session1/EGM_25Feb2019_S1_SergeiScherbov.pdf
2. Brown GC. Living too long, the current focus of medical research on increasing the quantity, rather than the quality, of life, is damaging our health and harming the economy. 2015.
3. https://www.who.int/news-room/fact-sheets/detail/dementia
4. https://www.medicinanarrativa.eu/wp-content/uploads/Remind-Portable-FINALE-compressed.pdf
5. https://www.ucl.ac.uk/news/2022/apr/pandemic-shielding-led-two-fold-increase-depressive-symptoms-older-people#:~:text=Older%20people%20who%20were%20shielding,according%20to%20researchers%20from%20UCL.
6. Leopardi G. I Canti. 1835.
7. https://onlinelibrary.wiley.com/doi/10.1002/hec.4613?af=R

Chapter 7
Where We Were and Are Now with Digital Health in Communication

The era we live in is post-contemporary, and philosopher Francesca Ferrando goes beyond this definition, calling it a posthumanism age [1]. It means that we overcome the anthropocentric humanistic approach, encompassing and even being threatened by the technological crafts of Artificial Intelligence (AI).

There is a philosophical stream called *Extropy*, originated by Max More in *The Principles of Extropy* [2]. This is an evolving framework of values and standards for continuously improving the human condition. Extropians believe that advances in science and technology will someday let people live indefinitely. An extropian may contribute to this goal by researching, developing, or volunteering to test new technology. Extropian thinking places a strong emphasis on rational thought and on practical optimism. According to More, these principles do not specify beliefs, technologies, or policies. Extropians share an optimistic view of the future, expecting considerable advances in computational power, life extension, nanotechnology and the eventual realization of indefinite lifespans and recovery through future advancements in biomedical technology such as, mind uploading (a process in which one's body/brain have been preserved through cryonics at temperatures below freezing). The term "*Extropy*" was invented on the principle of the opposition to Entropy, the eventual increase of chaos and energetic waste. This paradigm is also called transhumanism, very different from posthumanism, since in the former case, there is a continuous interchange between humans and technology to give meaning to lives in a world where every individual life is interconnected through technology not only to the present but also to our future.

The posthuman relationship existed before COVID-19 in places like Japan, the United States, the United Kingdom, China and other Western countries. It evoked a future in which humans could depend not on each other but on robots or other non-human entities. COVID-19 was a catalyst for the increased development of Digital Health, including telemedicine, teleconsultation, and telerehabilitation. In 2020, almost 60% of psychotherapy visits were done using Zoom,

Skype, and Teams platforms during the lockdown. In other fields, such as education, distance learning guaranteed the training program to move on (with the consequences we have seen in Chap. 4), but we could say that most of our activities were impacted by the digital reality. Smart working, home banking, home delivery, this digital quantic leap, that forcedly occurred during the pandemic is in healthcare and is here to stay. Organizations are now trying to find the Golden Ratio between being far but superficially connected and being near in full presence.

In the posthuman age, we do not know if the quote from Aristotle's "Politics," at the basis of our Western culture is still valid:

> A *Human being is, by nature, a social animal; an individual who is unsocial naturally and not accidentally is either beneath our notice or more than human. Society is something that precedes the individual. Anyone who cannot lead the common life or is so self-sufficient as not to need to, and therefore does not partake of society, is either a beast or a god.*

From a demographic point of view, Western countries are significantly ageing, with fragmented families, a considerable amount of lonely people and an essential need for caregiving. Our society is pushing the biomedical model rather than the biosocial, psychological, and spiritual model, in which the importance of human touch and bonding is paradigmatic. In a few words, we could say that there is a risk towards too many chronic illnesses taken care of by robots and too few vitalities coming out of human relationships in this social paradigm for the elderly—but even more than this, also in our civil society.

Nevertheless, hopefully, the eye-opening experience of COVID-19 brought back under light the need for human touch, as indicated by a unique study performed at the UCL [3]. Professor Aikaterini Fotopoulou from the UCL Division of Psychology and Language Sciences found that the quarantine period led people to crave touch more, but the extent of this craving varied depending on a person's early experiences of close relationships.

The researchers used an online survey (of around 1800 people) to test the effects of touch deprivation restrictions during the pandemic. They found that interpersonal and particularly intimate touch experiences are critical for mental health in times of distress and uncertainty.

The results revealed that people show more mood and anxiety symptoms when deprived of intimate touch. Those deprived of contact with people close to them reported increased perceptions of loneliness. The higher the number of days that people practiced social distancing, the more they wanted to experience touch, with the magnitude of this effect being large.

COVID-19 has taught us how much contact and touch are essential, scientifically demonstrating Aristotle's quote. After three years of pandemic, we know that we are collecting the broken pieces of the "pot" and trying to put them together using glue, gold, or whatever technique necessary.

Caregiving is a mix of actions and emotions: older people, ill people, and everybody who lives in a vulnerable situation may recover through this combined approach of facts of care and empathy.

Human contact is the most crucial thing for child development. Hugging is the first thing that allows bonding and establishes a sense of security in children. When we are ill, we regress to that time of seeking bonding and belonging to our people, clan, other human beings, or living beings. This is the body narrative; we must return to our ancestors' gestures not wasting time with too many words online. The body is there, the body speaks, and when it speaks, its language is more authentic than the said words.

We will examine robotics applications in caregiving for elderly people, remote doctors, and Italian research on telemedicine carried out in 2022, for ending up with the now unmissable Chat-GPT (July 2023, while writing).

7.1 Robot

The word *robot* comes from the Czech *robotnik* and means "forced working," or compulsory service. Are they only living in Asimov's science fiction book? No, they are already with us. According to the United Nations, the number of people 60 and older is expected to skyrocket to 2.1 billion in 2050. By 2030, according to the World Health Organization, 1 in 6 people in the world will be aged 60 years or over, and by 2050, the world's population of people aged 60 years and older will double (2.1 billion). The number of persons aged 80 or older is expected to triple between 2020 and 2050 to reach 426 million. At the same time, countless people regularly use technology, such as smartphones and Google Home, to enhance their lives.

The AARP (American Association of Retired People) is the USA's largest non-profit, nonpartisan organization dedicated to empowering Americans 50 and older to choose how they live as they age. *The iPad's elder-focused software is developed, and it can remind to take medicine and provide entertaining content and mind-stimulating puzzles. Their AI games are aimed at limiting the cognitive decay of Alzheimer's, celebrating Brain functionalities. It is joined with other "socially assistive" robots such as the Intuition Robotics', coaching and educating older US adults to good health.* "Socially assistive" robots can be helpful if patients are in the early stages of physical or cognitive decline.

Another therapeutic robot from Japan is named Paro, a "fake" seal, an advanced interactive robot. It allows the benefits of animal and pet therapy to be administered to patients in environments such as hospitals and extended care facilities where live animals cannot be admitted for safety reasons and logistical difficulties. Paro has five kinds of sensors: tactile, light, audition temperature, and posture sensor, with which it can perceive people and their environment. Paro can recognize light and dark, the direction of voice and words such as its name, greetings and praise. It works in the Japanese context as the result of a historical process in which robots were consciously designed to evoke positive feelings.

We might think about it as challenging to be exported in our culture; however, it was exported, and I would love to ask the reader whether to choose a fake friendly robot as a pet or a real animal, like a cat or a dog, which needs care. Studies with severely depressed people resulted from narratives of how pets were sometimes together with a small journey, the first steps to see the light after the tunnel.

Although looking like an oddity, Paro reached the UK, bypassing the transcultural Eastern and Western barriers, [4] where it is employed to care for people with Dementia. "Socially assistive" robots could replace the hard job of being a caregiver, which can be tedious, ghastly intimate and physically and emotionally exhausting. Caregiving time seems never-ending. The lives of caregivers, primarily low-income or unpaid women, are dramatically changed, together with the erosion of their self-realization. Caregivers' experiences are eroded by wanted or unwanted symbiosis with the elder or patient. An empathetic human caregiver is preferable to a robot. Still, due to an excessive burnout of caregivers, caregiving robots might be better than an unreliable or abusive person or a caregiver who gave himself/herself and eventually developed compassion fatigue.

The case of Mr. Quintana in the palliative care field (a pre-Covid but still very useful case):

Have you read the news? Do you know what's happened? What do you think about what happened in social media and WhatsApp chats? June 2019

I had not heard, nor was I particularly interested until I found myself watching the TV news: *"Robot doctor tells the patient he's going to die."* Even at this point, I felt no emotions. Still, then I watched the scene recorded by the granddaughter of Ernest Quintana, 78 years, a patient at a Hospital in Fremont, California, managed by Kaiser Permanente, an established and respected Health Maintenance Organization, which presents itself with these words on the homepage of their website in June 2019:

> Thrive your way. We'll take care of the rest. There are many ways to live healthily. Also, when you're a Kaiser Permanente member, many people work together to help you stay that way. Your doctor, specialists, and health plan are all part of one connected team —coordinating your care seamlessly, so you don't have to. It's how we do things faster, easier, and better—and help you live healthily.

With this slogan, on March 9, 2019, a robot appeared in the hospital room where the patient Ernest Quintana was lying, and through a video-link screen, a doctor appeared in a remote place to tell the patient, *"You might not make it home, you have no lungs left."* The granddaughter, Annalisa, who was present as caregiver, knew he was very ill, but she and her family had no idea of the extent up to this point. The one-way conversation continued with the Remote-Control Doctor informing the patient, who was not conscious, *"There is a risk that your breathing is too weak…we don't have an effective treatment, but I can give you comfort therapy, take off the oxygen mask and activate a morphine drip."*

Since the patient could not hear or comprehend, the granddaughter had the difficult task of translating into easy words the bad news and, unwittingly, did the doctor a favor by obtaining from the patient the legal consent needed to take away the oxygen mask and move to palliative sedation (euphemistically called comfort therapy) through morphine administration. Quintana died the next day, and the family was shocked by this chain of events.

Michelle Gaskill-Hames, senior vice-president of Kaiser Permanente Greater Southern Alameda County, called the situation highly unusual and said officials "regret falling short" of the patient's expectations, but said that telemedicine and teleconsultation is very effective and that they " ...*will use this as an opportunity to review how to improve the patient's experience with* tele-*video capabilities.*"

There was no outright admission of error—"falling short" meant simply being unable to satisfy the client, with the event labelled "as an opportunity" to continue with a practice that appears to have significant problems.

Well, if at the beginning I was only interested in the facts, looking at the whole process, I now must admit my surprise and annoyance with these facts during the pre-Covid age. Firstly, using a video link with a Remote Doctor looked like a dystopic science fiction movie. Unfortunately, it reminds us of the massive COVID-19 death toll between February and April 2020 in Europe, albeit here in this most recent pandemic case. Doctors were on the verge of tears because they had to take the "Remote Route," perceived as a non-human system for informing the family members of the death. The Quintana case was the analogy of 2001 Space Odyssey Stanley Kubrick movie, in which the computer HAL 9000 had to inform the spaceship captain that he would soon be dead. Also in this real case, the doctor was communicating a "death sentence," since it was not simply of a routine visit, with a possible change of therapy, and doctor and patient were not doing any telerehabilitation or teleconsultation: such a delicate communication about the imminent end of life was given in a virtual world, an "outer space," so far from reality.

The style of language used by the doctor, in this case, is like one learnt from the 0-1 binary code with which Computers and Robots work, possibly rude up to violent: Since active treatment is not working, we must move to "comfort therapy." The top of this absurd situation was achieved asking the question by the Doctor to the patient: *"Do you understand me?"* A question almost impossible to ask if the doctor was in the patient's room, in his proximity, gazing at his face, hands, body and condition.

He would never have asked this "rhetorical question" for two main reasons: the first is that being physically there, at the bedside, he would have in his eyes and hands much more detail of the complex picture of the conscious status of the patient (the doctor had in his hand simply an MRI lung image and not the patient's brain image) and secondly, the fact that unless one does not have mirror neurons, a developed empathetic human being would never ask such a question. Poor granddaughter Annalisa tried to translate the doctor's words, but her fumbling words to his grandfather were those of someone "over her pay grade": "your breathing will be stuck," no other words to add. She was put in an awkward, inhumane situation through no fault.

The management of Kaiser Permanente claimed that *many people work together to help you stay that way, healthy. Your doctor, specialists, and health plan are all part of one connected team*, but in this case, the patient was dying and *"Your doctor"* was somewhere lost in translation.

Telemedicine and teleconsultation are extraordinary tools for guaranteeing patient monitoring, especially in a home care setting or for specific purposes in a hospital, but not for replacing core visits. There are crucial moments which require an alignment between the doctor, the patient, and caregiver, if necessary. Such instances may include but are not limited to the communication of a diagnosis, treatment progress (whether "good" or "bad"), and to come to an agreement on a decision in the treatment, requiring communication in the diagnosis, as giving bad news and decision-making process. I think that this Mr. Quintana case is the quintessence of a tremendous violence against the dying man, against the caregiver and even against the poor doctors, embedded in such a broken system that forces the person to look after his patient in this unnatural way. Palliative care is where the physical encounter between carers and patients during end-of-life care is most important. It's the final salutation; grief has already begun.

Technology can be used in certain moments, and we have seen their extraordinary use during the COVID-19 pandemic, at least to bring a sort of continuity to chronic patients, to guarantee the correct administration of medication, and to avoid human errors with samples in the laboratory. Even in certain phases of surgery, it has been shown that a human eye as is always necessary to observe, perceive, understand, reflect and react to what is happening. Telemedicine might imply distance and loss of empathy. *If doctors are not well trained,* and of course, the case mentioned was that of a naive telemedical doctor with no digital empathic developed skills. This is why this event is, and will remain, a paradigmatic malpractice didactic case to be used by everyone in healthcare who wants to learn to become not a good carer but a poor carer.

7.2 Towards Alienation

In an essay on Tolkien, the author of *The Lord of the Rings*, which tried to summarize in a few lines the vastness of the literary works of the English novelist during the first half of the twentieth century, I was pleased to discover that the central message of his works is not the fight between Good and Evil, but the struggle between natural forces and those of industrialization and the creation of machines (today we would call them robots). The machine's ability to corrupt is visible not only in warfare and military conquest but also in everyday life, as it can remove something innately human and transform it into something dull and enervating. The dire implications of the machine are captured in Tolkien's Orcs. These creatures do not exist naturally but are bred by an evil power, out of the slime of the earth. They are deformed and ugly creatures whose hands are sometimes replaced with weapons. They seem to hate everyone, even themselves; they are alienated clones and take pleasure only in destroying and defiling. Tolkien suggests they make no beautiful things, perhaps because they cannot recognize beauty. They care only about efficiency and conquest and are driven by evil masters who rule through fear. On the other hand, we have the Ents in J. R. R. Tolkien's fantasy world, who closely resemble trees and have always been with us on this planet.

They are talking trees and appear in The Lord of the Rings as ancient shepherds of the forest and allies of the free peoples of Middle Earth. Ents are an old race, belonging to the most ancient natural realm, and will fight against the loss of souls produced on the earth by the Orcs and their chiefs. Death is such a natural embedded delicate moment that it should be honored, mourned, and supported with the respect given by the natural cycle of life and passing by. This is what humanities teaches. Now, more than ever before, after the COVID-19 in the Anthropocene age, looking at our skills to destroy the planet, and looking forward to achieving sustainable development goals, we might get back to the Ents and their strength to oppose the dumb arrival of some robots (not all)–the Orcs- are used to replace human beings in very delicate matters, where human touch is requested.

Now, try to think and feel. *What it would be like to be assisted by a caregiver robot? What could be the minimal requirements to allow a robot to be our caregiver? What do we think about pet therapy with Paro? What would it be like to receive violent human caregiving?* Finally, *would we define all these phenomena as utopian, extropian or dystopian?* Only some people could access the newest robot application, which would create further inequalities.

7.3 Developing a Wise Telemedicine

After having ingested these information and reflections on the use of AI, we wish to show the results of an Italian Research on Telemedicine performed by ISTUD in 2021-2022, "Effectiveness, efficiency and care humanizations with the use of telemedicine" [5].

Telemedicine and digital health are the transversal solutions promoted by the institutions (AGENAS, Ministry of Health and Regional Institutions) for the relaunch of the National Health System post- covid, being able to dispose of the substantial resources in the National Recovery and Resilience Plan (15.6 billion allocated for the "Health" mission of the Plan, of which 8.6 billion for innovation and digitalization and 7 billion for proximity networks, facilities and telemedicine for territorial assistance).

The ISTUD research on telemedicine aimed to understand the experience and narrative of people who used telemedicine and technological tools in general during the SARS-COV2 pandemic. From July 2021 to March 2022, 110 testimonies were collected involving all actors of the health ecosystem: patients, caregivers, health professionals, life science companies, researchers, and health policymakers.

Analyses of the narratives revealed numerous positive aspects of using technology to support medicine. One particularly striking output of the study was the ability to convey empathy even through the remote instrument; in many cases, compassion was experienced more in deferred time because, according to the doctors, *"being able to focus only on the face of the sick person helped connect with the patient's narratives and emotions."* Among the emerging problematic aspects is the impossibility of using telemedicine for first visits or emergencies, i.e. in cases where there is a need for real physical contact.

Questioning the humanization of technological tools and the need to take advantage of telemedicine opportunities is extremely important. Still, the starting question posed by Dr. Fabrizio Gervasoni, member of the Board of Directors of the Physicians Guild of Milan and Province, and Physiatrist at the Sacco-Fatebenefratelli Hospital is:

> *Will we doctors be able to remain clinical, to have contact with the patient, proximity with the patient, even in a setting such as telemedicine, where 'tele' represents a distance? The challenge is to be able to understand how, through doctors' languages, the perception of empathy with the patient can be maintained.*

This research, with 110 narratives with a prevalence of patients, doctors, caregivers, decision-makers, and healthcare companies, shows that empathy is a very present element; if one works on education in digital health, humanization remains, and patients feel listened to and understood even at a distance. From patients' narratives:

> *Initially, I was very skeptical: Being a great advocate of human contact, I believed that meeting my carer through a screen would be frustrating and less satisfying. I was wrong.*
>
> *The competence, thoroughness and even professionalism with which the doctor constructed the pathway resulted in a counselling that perfectly replicates those carried out in the Institute, and which I consider to be without flaws and/or criticalities.*
>
> Having several non-private health facilities where one can quickly turn to *"and not always having to resort to the private specialist, also because economic resources are limited, and not having to search for specialized facilities on the Internet"*.

Patients write about the de-materialization of the body:

> *Corporeality is very important; in fact, my carer's approach is to listen to one's inner self and body. It will be increasingly widespread, but much must be done to understand how to avoid dehumanizing care and digitalizing the human.*
>
> *I would need to be somewhat obliged to be waited on in a place, or at least to sign in. Even if only to be able to tell my employer that I really must go out for physiotherapy, or to not always be kidnapped by other urgencies.*
>
> *On the other hand, there is a lack of direct contact with the doctor.*
>
> *…human contact is basic for therapeutic purposes.*

From doctors' narratives:

> *The use of these new tools makes me feel greater comfort and agility in the intervention, even if I feel a lesser sensation of proxemics body proximity.*
>
> *Always useful but sometimes limited concerning certain relational and psychological dynamics typical of the cancer patient.*
>
> *…limited…both in seeing my patients in their entirety and in communicating not directly to people.*
>
> *Some of them, due to motor difficulties, prefer the teleconsultation, but we lose a range of information that is also useful to the therapeutic alliance, the emotional side.*

The "Zoom Gaze" is not as effective as seeing the whole body, as the doctors agreed. Health policy makers write:

> *…a hypothesis of the future to improve care and decrease inequalities. More cost-effective, greater access to care, an effort that will take several years and the training of health personnel.*

> It cannot be applied when the situation of the patient is such that it is not possible to connect, he/she lives alone, he (she does not have a caregiver, due to social, cultural conditions it is impossible.
>
> It is not the instrument that cannot be used in a circumstance, but the way, the standards of use. In other countries, it is also identified from the legal point of view. From a moral point of view, it cannot replace the doctor-patient relationship; the feasibility also depends on the systems. But there is a limit.

Fundamental is not to dehumanize and *"to ensure that the doctor-patient relationship remains relevant at all times, not only, unfortunately, as we often record from the narratives, when the patient is frail".*

The telemedicine tool is handy between one visit and the next; it is useful to support and sustain a chronic illness that needs continuous monitoring precisely to overcome the logistical and bureaucratic problems that public health has.

Among the actors involved, those who are the least satisfied with telemedicine and who have put up the most resistance are the caregivers, who are not only those who take care of the patient, providing physical and psychological assistance, but also must worry about the setting of the space, the organization of the light, the computer, the video camera, and in general the remote connection.

These results are self-evident, meaning that the quality of a relationship depends almost always on the people behind the screens, their soft skills for listening, creating a safe dialogue space, and "understanding" vulnerability and fragility, even from outer space. Intimacy in digital connection is possible and not a taboo anymore.

7.4 The Naissance of a New Paradigm: Chat GPT

It was December 2022, the first time I was told about Chat GPT: "What is it?" I asked, "Serious stuff, I was answered, not a game; try yourself to write a text." I registered and entered the words "Narrative Medicine," and I received a very elegant two-page text of clear and structured explained synthesis of what narrative medicine is. I searched for more recent information, browsing my autobiography and other scholars in the same field. Still, the very polite standard answer was, "I apologize; I cannot retrieve information after 2021," possibly because I was using the free version.

Chat GPT is an artificial intelligence chatbot developed by OpenAI and launched on November 30, 2022. It is notable for enabling users to refine and steer a conversation towards a desired length, format, style, detail level, and language. Successive prompts and replies are considered at each conversation stage as a context.

By January 2023, it had become the fastest-growing consumer software application, gaining over 100 million users. Some observers expressed concern over the potential of ChatGPT to displace or atrophy human intelligence and its potential to enable plagiarism or fuel misinformation.

ChatGPT was released as a freely available research preview, but OpenAI now operates the service on a freemium model due to its popularity. It allows users on its free tier to access the GPT-3.5-based version.

ChatGPT was built with a safety system against harmful content: sexual abuse, verbal and physical violence, racism, sexism, and other discriminatory content. Chat GPT, besides some inaccurate information, has a very kind, empathic and warm narrative genre, rejecting any rude text.

7.5 Chat GPT in the Healthcare System

The promise of Chat GPT was also tested in the healthcare sector, and results were published in April 2023 in a prestigious Journal as JAMA (6). How do doctors inform their patients about their diagnosis? What is the level of accuracy? And how are you empathetic with the situation?

The study's premise was this: "Virtual healthcare has caused a surge in patient messages concomitant with more work and burnout among healthcare professionals. Artificial intelligence (AI) assistants could potentially aid in creating answers to patient questions by drafting responses that clinicians could review." The objective was to evaluate the ability of an AI chatbot assistant (ChatGPT) to provide quality and empathetic responses to patient questions.

In a cross-sectional study, a public and nonidentifiable database of questions from a public social media forum (Reddit's r/AskDocs) was used to randomly draw 195 exchanges from October 2022 where a verified physician responded to a public question. Chatbot responses were generated by entering the original question into a fresh session (without prior questions being asked) on December 22 and 23, 2022. The original question and anonymized and randomly ordered physician and chatbot responses were evaluated in triplicate by a team of licensed healthcare professionals. Evaluators chose "which response was better". They judged both "the quality of information provided" (*very poor, poor, acceptable, sound,* or *very good*) and "the empathy or bedside manner provided" (*not empathetic, slightly empathetic, moderately empathetic, empathetic,* and *very empathetic*). Mean outcomes were ordered on a 1 to 5 scale and compared between the chatbot and physicians.

Of the 195 questions and responses, evaluators preferred chatbot responses to physician responses in 78.6% (95% CI, 75.0–81.8%) of the 585 evaluations. Mean (IQR) physician responses were significantly shorter than chatbot responses (52 [17–62] words vs. 211 [168–245] words; $t = 25.4$; $P < 0.001$). Chatbot responses were rated of significantly higher quality than physician responses ($t = 13.3$; $P < 0.001$). The proportion of responses rated as *good* or *very good* quality (≥ 4), for instance, was higher for chatbot than physicians (chatbot: 78.5%, 95% CI, 72.3–84.1%; physicians: 22.1%, 95% CI, 16.4–28.2%). This amounted to a 3.6 times higher prevalence of *good* or *excellent* quality responses for the chatbot. Chatbot responses were also rated significantly more empathetic than physician responses ($t = 18.9$; $P < 0.001$). The proportion of responses rated *empathetic* or *very empathetic* (≥ 4) was higher for chatbot than for physicians (physicians: 4.6%, 95% CI, 2.1–7.7%; chatbot: 45.1%, 95% CI, 38.5–51.8%; physicians: 4.6%, 95% CI, 2.1–7.7%). This amounted to a 9.8 times higher prevalence of *empathetic* or *very empathetic* responses for the chatbot.

A chatbot generated quality and empathetic responses to patient questions online in this cross-sectional study. *"Further exploration of this technology is warranted in clinical settings, such as using a chatbot to draft replies that physicians could edit. Randomized trials could further assess whether using AI assistants might improve responses, decrease clinician burnout, and improve patient outcomes"* [6].

The clinical setting is very different from an open forum in virtual mode. In daily practice, doctors and patients are physically there, with their personalities, competencies, and emotions. Therefore, translating these conclusions to real-life care settings would take time and effort. However, these results may draw the route for the ecosystem to create between AI and Health Care Providers. Beyond the authors' conclusion of using AI-Chat-GPT to reduce burnout, burnout is reduced when more nourishing and empathetic relationships are created with the patients. It is the narrative part that Chat-GPT covers with the longer answers, that the real-life doctors are rejecting somehow, as "sons and daughters of EBM." The reductionist model of biomedicine also shrinks the language possibility and the empathy skills. This result looks very odd since we would have been most likely expecting more accuracy but less relationship using AI.

Why these results? We said, "sons and daughters of an EBM-cracy," of lessons of detachment from patients, with the teaching of a "clinical gaze, which should not look into patients' eyes". In which system? In health care organizations strangled by continuous downsizing, constrained to a hyper- efficiency; this poisons the ecosystem made of healthcare professionals and patients, and increase the risk of rude answers, verbal violent replies and in an escalation, physical violence. Soft skills or humanities, ironically, are called non-technical skills, so the very competencies so essential to develop are robbed of a proper name, in a very ignorant and short-sighted way, ignoring that there is a technique to develop empathy, communication and teamwork. The outcome of this choice of terms is that doctors while updating their competence, will read preferably only technical papers, neglecting the other humanities papers, not perceiving the facts that humanities and techniques are intertwined to provide good care -diagnosis is also an art, not just a mere technical process. Behind the chosen words, there is a narrative competence.

If we don't repair now and urgently, the human touch of Doctors and Carers will be replaced by Artificial Intelligence that will never suffer from compassion fatigue but always show lovely compassion without the needs of human beings.

7.6 Practice Time

7.6.1 The Case of Technology Replacing Doctors' Human Actions in Diagnosis and Intervention

Researchers at the John Radcliffe Hospital in Oxford, England, developed an Artificial Intelligence (AI) diagnostic system that's more accurate than doctors at diagnosing heart disease at least 80% of the time.

At Harvard University, researchers created a "smart" microscope that can detect potentially lethal blood infections. The AI-assisted tool was trained on a series of 100,000 images from 25,000 slides treated with dye to make the bacteria more visible. The AI system can already sort those bacteria with a 95% accuracy rate. A study from Showa University in Yokohama, Japan, revealed that a new computer-aided endoscopic system could show signs of potentially cancerous growths in the colon with 94% sensitivity, 79% specificity, and 86% accuracy [7].

In some cases, researchers found that AI can outperform human physicians in diagnostic challenges that require a quick judgment call, such as determining if a lesion is cancerous. In one study, published in December 2017 in JAMA, deep learning algorithms [8] were able to diagnose better metastatic breast cancer than human radiologists. While human radiologists may do well with limited time to review cases, in the real world (especially in high-volume, quick-turnaround environments like emergency rooms), a rapid diagnosis could make the difference between life and death for patients. However, this is familiar since technology has always been an aid in helping doctors to formulate a diagnosis.

With which words should doctors communicate information about the diagnosis? Will their words be chosen with wisdom and empathy, or will the robot take this over to have fewer defensive problems? Please remember the empathic results of Chat-GPT.

Let's move to surgery:

Surgical robots are an extension of the human surgeon, who controls the device from a nearby console. One of the more ambitious procedures claimed to be the first-ever globally occurred in Montreal in 2010. It was the first in-tandem performance of a surgical robot and a robot anesthesiologist, with the nick name as *McSleepy:* this AI robot can be thought of as a sort of humanoid anesthesiologist that thinks like an anesthesiologist, analyses biological information, and constantly adapts its own behavior, even monitoring and recognizing malfunction. The data gathered on the procedure reflects the impressive performance of Mc Sleepy and other robotic doctors.

In 2015, MIT performed a retrospective analysis of FDA data to assess the safety of robotic surgery. The report noted that *most procedures were successful and had no problems.* However, complication events in more complex surgical areas like cardiothoracic surgery were "significantly higher" than in gynecology and general surgery. It means that a future career is guaranteed for doctors and surgeons who must perform very complicated procedures. Still, in terms of sustainability, for secure operations, despite patients screaming and searching for the human touch, from an economic and even safety point of view, the "Dr. Knife" robot is here [9].

As a doctor, future doctor, or other healthcare professional (HCP), how do you envision that a robot might replace your activity? How do you think it will happen, and what do you think that the doctors and HCP will tend to act more in their role? Please take your time write at least five attitudes for your profession, the so-called five good reasons for waking up in the morning.

7.6.2 The Doctor-Engineer Emerging Role

There is an academic program between Hunimed, the faculty of Medicine at Humanitas University and Politecnico, the Faculty of Engineering [10]. The aim is the creation of a hybrid profession, a Doctor-Engineer. This merge could be very beneficial to make sure that doctors can contribute to creating new technologies. Currently, this is co-creation process carried out by doctors, biomedical engineers, and IT experts. Here, a new discipline is created, embracing only technical skills.

Alas, Humanities are once more steps behind, they remain neglected in the shadow of technical skills. Instead, I would propose the rise of a new course in medicine joined with Philosophy to create a new hybrid, the Philosopher-Doctor. Alternatively, a Humanist Doctor, skilled also with robotic knowledge.

Since we know that Extropy will continue, human thoughts, feelings and words are desired and must be preserved although blended with technology. An investment in creating the engineer-doctor is worth the survival of the "doctor species." Given the way that most of the faculties of Medicine teaches the art of providing care through algorithms, this venture is a tactic, but I cannot predict how strategic it will be in the long run. A new paradigm of health care would have been represented by letting the robots do their job, constantly improving under the AI experts, including doctors, philosophers, economists, anthropologists, psychologists, nurses, caregivers, patients, and individuals on a multidisciplinary team. Human careers could avoid the threat of losing their job by focusing more on existential issues, communications, emotions, words, and gestures, that is, the Humanities for Health.

I dream an interdisciplinary teaching where STEM (Science, Technology, Engineering and Mathematics) and SHAPE (Social Sciences, Humanities and the Arts for People and the Economy/Environment) disciplines are woven together.

We must not run the risk of being overwhelmed by the technology we could create, but keep our focus fixed on helping the human being to flourish. Let us refrain from using the mindset "either humanist or technologist," but "both humanist and technologist," bearing in mind that humanism is embedded in every technology.

7.6.2.1 Reading Isaac Azimov's *I, Robot*

Isaac Azimov, a clairvoyant of robotics, wrote his extraordinary series of fiction novels *I, Robot*, in which he is the first to mention *Robopsychology*, the study of the personalities and behavior of intelligent machines. *Robbie*, written in 1940, has an exquisite plot. In the year 1982, a mute robot, Robbie, is owned by the Weston family. He serves as a nanny for their daughter, Gloria.

Mrs. Weston has become concerned about how a robot might affect Gloria's still-developing social skills and that he might malfunction and harm her. Gloria prefers Robbie's company to that of other children. Mr. Weston returns Robbie to the factory, and to justify Robbie's disappearance, Gloria's parents claim that he had, for no reason, "walked away." They, instead, replace him with a *collie dog* called Lightning.

The effort fails. Gloria, missing Robbie, stops enjoying life. Her mother thinks it would be impossible for Gloria to forget the robot while surrounded by the places where they once played. Mrs. Weston convinces her husband to take them to New York, where he happens to work. Gloria gets the wrong idea, optimistically thinking that they have gone to the city in search of Robbie.

Among other tourist attractions, the Westons visit the Museum of Science and Industry where Gloria sneaks away to see a "Talking Robot," a *computer* that takes up the whole room. It can answer questions posed to it verbally by visitors. Gloria asks the machine if it knows how to find Robbie, "a robot... just like you," she says. The computer, unable to comprehend the question, breaks down.

Mr. Weston approaches his wife with the idea of touring a robot factory. Gloria can then see robots as inanimate objects, not "people." During the tour, Mr. Weston asks to see a room where robots make other robots, where it just so happens that one of the robot assemblers is Robbie. Gloria runs in front of a moving vehicle in her eagerness to get to her friend but is rescued by Robbie. Both parents agree that the two friends can stay together when Robbie saves Gloria's life.

Here are the famous three laws of robotics:

First Law
A robot may not injure a human being or, through inaction, allow a human being to come to harm.
Second Law
A robot must obey the orders given to it by human beings except where such orders would conflict with the First Law.
Third Law
A robot must protect its existence as long as such protection does not conflict with the First or Second Law.

How far we have come together, reader! From the possible evil inherent in, the one Tolkien feared in his *Lord of the Rings*, to experiencing the benefits of having a robotic pet, and the awe we may experience as patients tell us that they feel more listened to when they are visited through telemedicine and that doctors confirm this as they reported increased focused on the video in order to grasp every possible detail. Furthermore, we assessed with both fear and wonder how Chat GPT was said to be, 9 times out of 10, more empathetic in an open forum than doctors in the flesh. And finally, we shared Isaac Azimov's vision of the potential goodness of these systems, robots as caregivers, and nurses, because all these systems are designed to take care of the human being by our evolved brain, that of the frontal lobes, of co-operation, and the mirror neurons of empathy, setting rules to contain and limit possible neglect, harm and violence.

References

1. Ferrando F. Posthumanism, transhumanism, antihumanism, metahumanism, and new materialisms: differences and relations. Existenz. 2013;8(2):26–32.
2. https://web.archive.org/web/20131015142449/http:/extropy.org/principles.htm

References

3. Mohr MV, Kirsch LP, Fotopoulou A. Huge experience with COVID-19 brought back under light the need for human touch. R Soc Open Sci. 2021.
4. https://www.brighton.ac.uk/research-and-enterprise/groups/healthcare-practice-and-rehabilitation/research-projects/the-paro-project.aspx.
5. https://www.medicinanarrativa.eu/la-telemedicina-nella-pratica-clinica-e-nella-ricerca-tra-efficacia-ed-umanizzazione-delle-cure
6. Ayers JW, et al. Comparing physician and artificial intelligence chatbot responses to patient questions posted to a public social media forum. JAMA. 2023;183(6):589–96.
7. Mori Y, et al. Computer-aided diagnosis for colonoscopy. Endoscopy. 2017;49(8):813–9.
8. Bejnordi BE, et al. Diagnostic assessment of deep learning algorithms for detection of lymph node metastases in women with breast cancer. JAMA. 2017;318(22):2199–210.
9. https://futurism.com/ai-medicine-doctor
10. https://www.ilsole24ore.com/art/a-milano-nasce-medico-ingegnere-doppia-laurea-politecnico-e-humanitas-AC2r3YN

Chapter 8
Violence of Power in the Role Status, Time and Size: Finding the Right Words, Timing and Dimension

Off with their heads!—Queen of Hearts,
I am late! I am late! For a very important appointment!
No time to say 'Bye, bye'! I'm late. I'm late, I'm late!—White Rabbit
Alice in Wonderland, Lewis Carroll

Almost all of us are familiar with the "Un-Birthday," the cruelty of the Queen of Hearts, and the Cheshire Cat of Alice in Wonderland. Since the given name is "Wonderland," and since Lewis Carroll was a mathematician, we might say that in this "wonderland kingdom," there are all possible degrees of freedom for the oddities to come true.

However, zooming past some topics of this novel, we come to understand that each character is a representation of a different mental illness: Little Alice suffers from Hallucinations and Personality Disorders; the White Rabbit from Generalized Anxiety Disorder; the Cheshire Cat has schizophrenia, as he disappears and reappears distorting reality around him, and subsequently, driving other characters in the story to madness. The Queen of Hearts is affected by egotism and narcissism; the hookah-smoking Caterpillar is consumed by drug addiction, and the Mad Hatter, simply by madness, repeating in an obsessive-compulsive way, for 10 years at 6 p.m. the celebration of our beloved Un-birthday. He is stuck there, with no sense of time, as he is gets older and older.

What about the Cards? They are just servants, there to obey, representations of depersonalization and codependency. Reading on the Red Queen's "constant orders for beheadings,"

8.1 The Risk of Narcissistic Disorder in Health Care Provider

> *"I see!" said the Queen, who had meanwhile been examining the roses. "Off with their heads!" 'and the procession moved on, three of the soldiers remaining behind to execute the unfortunate gardeners, who ran to Alice for protection.*
> *"You shan't be beheaded!" said Alice, and she put them into a large flowerpot that stood nearby. The three soldiers wandered about for a minute, looking for them, and then quietly marched off after the others.*
> *"Are their heads off?" shouted the Queen.*
> *"Their heads are gone if it pleases, your Majesty!" the soldiers shouted.*

The Narcissistic Queen of Hearts is the opposite of what a Heartful and Caring Queen should be. These lines are dedicated to the adventure of examining the level of Narcissistic disorders in healthcare providers.

A prospective cross-sectional study within multiple departments of a UK secondary care teaching hospital titled [1], "Mirror mirror on the ward, who's the most narcissistic of them all? Pathologic personality traits in health care," was conducted. A total of 248 healthcare professionals participated, and 159 members of the general population were recruited as a comparison group. Three personality traits—narcissism, Machiavellianism and psychopathy—were measured through the validated self-reported personality questionnaires Narcissistic Personality Inventory (NPI), MACH-IV and the Levenson Self-Report Psychopathy Scale (LSRP), respectively. The results showed that healthcare professionals scored significantly lower on narcissism, Machiavellianism and psychopathy (mean scores 12.0, 53.0 and 44.7, respectively) than the general population ($p < 0.001$). Within the cohort of medical professionals, surgeons expressed significantly higher levels of narcissism ($p = 0.03$, mean NPI score 15.0). This means that healthcare professionals expressed low levels of dark triad personality traits. The suggestion that healthcare professionals are avaricious and untrustworthy may be refuted, albeit surgeons might reach the levels of other non-health-related professions. Despite these findings, surgeons are becoming increasingly attracted to the Medical Humanities [1]. So, we are sometimes biased by our prejudice. However, there are other realities around the world that need to be spoken out.

Leanne Rowe was appointed Chairman of Nexus Hospitals in December 2019 and brings a strong background of leadership roles within the healthcare sector. She has received many prominent national awards for her service in healthcare. Having also worked as a rural GP for 25 years, Rowe has developed a deep insight into the private and public healthcare systems. Rowe currently holds board positions with the Medical Indemnity Protection Society (MIPS), MIPS insurance, and Japara Health Care, and presides over Medical Panels in Victoria, which involves chairing meetings of surgeons and physicians of many subspecialties to provide court determinations. She is a member of the Royal Australian College of General Practitioners and a Northwestern Primary Care Network member. She has written extensively on mental health, and her particular interest in workforce health provides an awareness of the importance of caring for clinicians and other staff and the positive impact this has on patient outcomes.

I attach her brief professional biography because, in a certain way, her statements will become helpful for describing a story of verbal and behavioral violence (not physical) that I witnessed, his nickname is Dr. King of Hearts—"Heads off."

Dr. Rowe writes:

> *How is it possible that endemic bullying persists in medicine despite a Senate inquiry, viral social media campaigns, doctor education, incident reporting and other initiatives to improve awareness, mutual respect and medical culture?*
>
> *Sometimes, we can blame health system issues, such as medical workforce shortages, lack of funding and unsafe hours. Still, in other cases, we must take collective responsibility for failing to hold individual doctors to account for their damaging behaviors.*
>
> *Most doctors readily change after being counselled about poor social skills, rudeness, bullying, sexual harassment, discrimination or racism. But others refuse to accept they have a problem and risk damaging their reputation, position, career, or accreditation. Why would doctors do this? And why is it so difficult for others to call them out and intervene effectively?*
>
> *One of the reasons may be due to narcissistic personality disorder (NPD).... In my experience of working in clinical and board leadership roles across many different medical workplaces for nearly three decades, doctors with untreated NPD may manifest bullying behaviors in a number of ways.*
>
> *Fundamentally, a doctor with NPD is arrogant, feels entitled and believes others have a problem. In subtle or not-so-subtle ways, they let other colleagues know they are "special," exaggerating their exceptional skills in patient diagnosis and management. Patients often adore them as they also inflate their achievements in their consulting rooms while making derogatory comments about the clinical management of other doctors. Consequently, a doctor with NPD may seem charming on the surface and have many admiring followers. Generous one day and dismissive or aloof the next, they justify their quick temper as necessary to keep other doctors on their toes and uphold a high patient care standard.*
>
> *To avoid being reported, doctors with NPD may slowly undermine their victims with repetitive nit-picking and sarcasm.... Intermittent stonewalling and private taunting are also tough to prove."*

The results of UK and Australia research are hopefully inconsistent, or better some are showing heartful Kings and Knights and Queens in the study conducted in the UK, but another one carried out in Australia produced the opposite result. This means that further research is warranted, but also, that this is a poor point of interest, since there are so few publications about this search topic. Personalities of Health Care Providers are not a priority to be studied in funded research, and we have to remind that Health Care Professionals are those who take care and cure people in their fragility and vulnerability times.

8.1.1 Dr. King of Hearts

In a recent Zoom meeting on narrative medicine research in neurology scheduled from 5 p.m. to 7 p.m. with all highly qualified specialists in a particular subject, Dr. King of Hearts, a very prestigious doctor with a skyrocket Impact Factor of

International publications, joined the meeting later at 5.30 p.m., not having time to saying hello to the others but boasting said, "I cannot stay here until midnight" with a very rude verbal and nonverbal language. While we were discussing on narrative texts, he switched the conversation to criticizing the belonging to a political party, completely going off-topic. We all have been condescending about his time constraint request; however, on every slide shown, he perceived something "untrue, fake or false." I was chairing the online meeting and replied in the kindest way I could (I remember my inner dialogue, *stay calm whatever might happen first, one step back,* using the first rule of nonviolent communication). I had to repeatedly remind the group that we are ambassadors of the written texts of patients, caregivers, and doctors, and that this study was not Evidence-Based Medicine, and it was not our intention at all to replace the EBM methodology with Narrative Medicine.

Regardless, Dr. King of Hearts continued attacking the research, wasting his time and our time. While trying to follow the rules of nonviolent communication, observing, and staying on the facts, and keeping it under control, I asked, "Please, could you read the authentic narratives?" This request was perceived as a further insult by his side. At that very moment, I received a message on WhatsApp from a colleague: "Leave it. He is a psychopath; everyone knows it in our scientific community." I knew in advance that he was not a handyman, but I could not even imagine that this kind of violence, with such rude words, and in a professional meeting, could come from this person. A few minutes later in the Zoom meeting, he declared, very annoyed, *"I am labelled as insensitive and not empathic."* I replied using the calmest, firmest, most docile voice I could muster, *"No one ever said that"* and he ended the conversation by saying, *"I don't want to be treated as a stupid."*

I reinforced this message in the public chat, generalizing the message: *"No one here in this meeting is calling anybody insensitive; no one here is calling anybody stupid."* After 5 min, Dr. King of Hearts quit the meeting, not even saying a final goodbye. After he quit, the atmosphere became lighter; people started to contribute again, praising the research and finding room for improvement. A very fruitful conversation, and we ended in time. One day later, we received excuses from a couple of people from members of his equipe for his behavior: these excuses were not needed, even if they were appreciated.

I was astonished that this man bullied a community of high-quality specialists and by inevitably silencing people: I do not want to understand the deep roots of this behavior, and perhaps he had a past which may justify part of it; however, as Leanne Rowe was writing, he might never attend a counselling course or try to understand the reason for his "violence."

I'm uncomfortable writing these lines because I would love to report only good things from the healthcare setting, especially my personal experience. Nevertheless, I felt the need to write about this event because there is a limit that we should not trespass. We, empathetic people, including you readers, otherwise I doubt you would be now reading these lines, tend to accept everyone's behavior. Though this tendency may have good intention, the lack of respect towards the work done, the other's culture, the other's feelings cannot be permitted, at least in a professional environment. Wonderland is a terrible place sometimes, not only inhabited by kind people but also tyrants, who will never seek a cure and will manipulate even the smartest people to behave as the Cards in Alice Wonderland, with vanished bodies and minds.

I also promised stories counterbalancing this behavior. They come from the parallel charts (reflective writings from doctors) written by his colleagues and peers. As a matter of fact, they write regarding the very project objectives discussed during this meeting. These are stories of humble, curious, motivated, competent doctors who wish to learn something new every day, describing their relationship with their patients affected by a very invalidating neurological condition.

> *Taking care of this person was...*
> *"It has been a great human and professional challenge."*
>> *It has been, yet another challenge brought against a little-known disease, and with the difficulties of the first months, I would say first year and more of treatment. I had and have the knowledge that I can steer the boat to port without major damage;*
> *"It makes me proud and satisfied to do my job"*
> *"I feel it as a serious responsibility, and it has been an opportunity for growth in my professional path."*
> And in the end, *"The experience of writing the parallel chart was..."*
> *"Pleasant"*
> *"Writing was Reflecting on the patient's experience and my own."*
> *"Lovely"*
> *"I love to write about positive experiences of redemption and courage."*
> *"Complex but stimulating"*
> *"Attractive, looking at me and this girl from the outside."*
> *"Liberating"*
> *"Epic reflection"*
> *"Strange. Liberating"*
> *"New and complicated experience"*
> *"Liberating"*
> *"It is not an insignificant experience, an incentive to remember."*

These were excerpts shown on the day of that "memorable" meeting, and as we can see, doctors full of zest, passion, and competence who embraced the reflective writing adventure. And, with the utmost surprise, our narrative medicine research in this particular field of neurology—(I cannot mention for privacy of the whole process)— was published after the first submission by a prestigious scientific journal.

8.2 No Time to Say "Hello"

The constant rush is also violent, as very well expressed by the White Rabbit: "no time to say hello"—Alice will remark it in the novel. Much in the same way, Dr. King of Hearts "could not stay until midnight," being engaged in so many other, "more valuable" things. However, I'm much more condescending in this case, thinking that the rudeness of linear time and how we handle our calendar, packing it with too many activities, is an illness of our times.

What is the impact of shortening the visit with patients, saving time? In a study which explored the length of stay with prescription appropriateness by primary care physicians, published in JAMA in 2023, the authors found the following, somehow expected, results [2]. It was a cross-sectional study that used data from electronic health record systems in primary care offices across the US to analyze adult primary care visits occurring in 2017. Analysis was conducted from March 2022 through January 2023.

Regression analyses were used to quantify the association between patient visit characteristics and visit length and the association between visit length and potentially inappropriate prescribing decisions, including inappropriate antibiotic prescriptions for upper respiratory tract infections, co-prescribing of opioids and benzodiazepines for painful conditions, and medications that were potentially inappropriate for older adults. The inappropriate prescription was based on the Beers criteria set by the American Geriatrics Society and reviewed every three years; they are very general and should be tailored to every visited patient, but they represent a compass. The criteria consist of a list of medications to avoid if you're over 65 years old, not in a hospice or a palliative care setting. The list also includes information about specific health conditions, and which combinations of medications to avoid since they cause dangerous side effects. All rates were estimated using physician-fixed effects and were adjusted for patient and visit characteristics.

This study included 8,119,161 primary care visits on 4,360,445 patients (56.6% women) performed by 8091 primary care physicians; 7.7% of patients were Hispanic, 10.4% were non-Hispanic Black, 68.2% were non-Hispanic White, 5.5% were another race and ethnicity, and 8.3% had missing race and ethnicity. Longer visits were more complex (i.e., more diagnoses recorded and/or more chronic conditions coded). After controlling for scheduled visit duration and measures of visit complexity (such as, age, whether they were insured by the public health system or lacking private health insurance), it was noted that Hispanic and non-Hispanic Black patients had shorter visits. For each additional minute of visit length, the likelihood that a visit resulted in an inappropriate antibiotic prescription changed by −0.11 percentage points (95% CI, −0.14 to −0.09 percentage points) and the likelihood of opioid and benzodiazepine co-prescribing changed by −0.01 percentage points (95% CI, −0.01 to −0.009 percentage points). Visit length is inversely associated with inappropriate prescribing among older adults (0.004 percentage points; 95% CI, 0.003–0.006 percentage points). *Shorter visit length was associated with a higher likelihood of inappropriate antibiotic prescribing for patients with upper respiratory tract infections and co-prescribing opioids and benzodiazepines for patients with painful conditions. These findings suggest visiting scheduling and quality of prescribing decisions in primary care.*

In conclusion, reading through all this numbers, given the deep racial and status inequities of care, there is an urgent call for equity and time for the publicly insured, Hispanic, and non-Hispanic Black patients, compared to the White patients and those with private insurance, which benefit from a more extended time. The researchers do not propose an optimal timeframe for a visit but highlights the need to address structured racism.

> *Maybe the White rabbit did not want to say hello to Alice just because she, in his opinion, was a meaningless child. Better to go to the Mad Hatter, who offered at six o'clock a nice cup of tea with biscuits.*—Between the lines.

Many studies have focused on the duration of doctors 'visits, with average results of 17 min in the years before 2020. In a study performed on primary care, evaluating the time to topics, patients who initiated the visit speaking about essential life topics for them, were not listened anymore by the doctors. This may suggest that physicians did not view those topics as being as significant as the patients did or, in a deeper thinking, that they were feeling powerless when patients behind the disease, were starting to open up about their illness and way of living. Similarly, physicians talked much less with patients when patients showed mood problems, also with body language. It raises a question about whether physicians feel disinclined to engage patients who appear depressed or anxious [3]. So, it's not only a matter of time, but also, a *"Weltanschauung mindset."* Are doctors equipped to listen to patient biographies, with the ups and downs, the pathography? This is why narrative medicine stands for teaching and embracing the narrative posture able to identify the speaking persons, the significant topics, and put in the background the details at that moment not necessary for the people to be cured.

A phenomenon of further time compression is taking place. The 17 min, in the narratives reported by the doctors themselves, are more likely now to be restricted to 10 min. In Europe, it is, on average, around 10–12 min, 9 in the United Kingdom, 12 in Germany, and 15 in France. Italy is not on the list but estimates by the Italian Society of General Medicine and the World Health Organization assume a visiting time of between 9 and 12 min. Typically, the patients are the first to complain about the brevity of doctor's visits and lengthy waitlists, then doctors become exasperated by this diagnostic and clinical rush that poses problems in understanding the patient's biographical context. The doctors know that if the policies on visit timeframe are not changed, they will be trapped in a *rabbit hole* with poor escape possibilities.

8.3 Tea-Time and The Rabbit Hole

Six o'clock, meaning tea-time, imprisons the characters of Alice in Wonderland for ages, stuck in that tea party. There are at least two meanings of time: a former, which runs ("I have to go," "I have to do," "I have to paint the white roses to become red to please the Queen," "no time to say hello"). On the other hand, there is a latter, hidden time, which is still: people are repeating the same scene, having the same role—as the ritual of the teatime for the Un-birthday party, where the invited are not even able to drink their cup of tea. Of course, time ran curiously in Wonderland because it was simply a dream. Another thing to remember is that when Alice wakes up from the dream, it is teatime, too.

As in Alice's novel, the doctors and healthcare providers might be imprisoned by the never-ending set of the same rules and protocols, despite every person they meet being unique. By applying the same checklist carefully, focusing on the disease, the HCP risks losing the beauty of "subjectivity" and "intimacy" with patients. They might enter in a "rabbit hole," which I use as a metaphor to describe burnout. Alice falls into the rabbit hole because she chases a white rabbit with pink eyes, because she saw the rabbit checking a pocket watch. Today, we use this term for spending too much time on something or getting too involved.

The rabbit hole is like an existential tunnel we must face in our personal and professional lives. Alice ends up in Wonderland in a depersonalized way. After entering the rabbit hole, she has to find the correct dose of "eat me" and "drink me" to recompose herself, and the hope of these lines is that every healthcare provider could find the right amount, wherever they are. My hope is that they would not invade others' rooms (as Alice did), and not disappear (also as Alice did), finding the right balance in midst of violence, impoliteness, and a shortage of time.

8.4 Practice Time

8.4.1 Reading of Patients' Violence Against Health Care Providers. Expanding Our Point of View

Violence is a relatively vague term with several meanings and interpretations. In the healthcare setting, violence may present itself as a verbal or physical attack by patients or visitors. In some cases, it could be verbal aggression (shouting, offences and threats), physical assault, and harassment.

Violence in healthcare is a critical worldwide issue. In a 2017 Assessment of Occupational Injuries and Illnesses, the Bureau of Labor and Statistics reports that healthcare workers are five times more likely to experience violence on the job than the average American worker [4].

In the US, gender and age are among the strongest predictors of violent behavior. Men younger than 35 are the highest offenders of violence against healthcare professionals. I choose not to invest some much time reviewing sociodemographic data, although one noteworthy finding is that lower the education level was correlated with a higher risk of violence. Nonetheless, there are many organizational and structural issues in the Healthcare System, for instance absurdly long waiting times, and a lack of security personnel. Patient areas being open to anyone are unfortunately the highest contributing place where violence occurs. Other contributing factors include:

- Lack of metal detectors.
- Delayed response time by security.

8.4 Practice Time

- Working between 7 p.m. to 7 a.m.
- Being alone with the patient or visitor.
- Lack of violence prevention training.
- Working long hours and night shifts.

Also, in Italy, from an institutional report of INAIL, violence and attacks on healthcare professionals are reported. These are very insidious since, as the institute says, they are related to a sort of "acquisitive pretension" on the part of the insured/technopathic person due to his/her belief that he "deserves" a certain service. In this dimension, healthcare workers may not be seen as allies but antagonists.

In US, the highest incidences reported are from paramedics, emergency departments, and inpatient psychiatric facilities. In 2016, healthcare workers made up 69% of all reported workplace violent injuries, according to the Bureau of Labor and Statistics. In Italy, from 2020 to 2022, in 70% of the cases of aggression were against women, 64% were employees of hospitals and nursing homes, and 80% were workers in residential and non-residential social care facilities. The offenders were mainly patients between the ages of 30 and 50, and the perpetrators of violence tend to be male. The patient's health was also a possible cause: severe mental disorders, substance use disorders, or cognitive impairments may make a patient more physically violent, whereas verbal aggression is more commonly observed in patients without these clinical characteristics [5]. The authors conclude their research by commenting that these events are not merely the outcome of a poor HCP-patient relationship. Still, they originate due to three external "layers" that they call "Business, Community and Society." Change is possible when facing it at a systemic level.

In Italy, where the outcome is the same with an increase in patient violence against HCP, the already exhausted NHS, with the turmoil of the pandemic, resulted in a poor organization of work characterized by staff shortages, excessive overtime, a low number of rest days and days off work. The gender gap has widened with significant salary differences; many senior staff have been called back into service, and junior teams have been called to new roles without sufficient preparation and specific sectoral experience.

This led to inevitable burnout and repercussions on the quality of care. The postponement of non-urgent services also created a backlog of medical care, with palliatives such as telemedicine, without the necessary literacy in the new method, together with all the medical-legal burdens that such services inevitably carry.

In a healthy organization driven by efficacy and quality, and not by brutalist efficiency, this risk of violence from patients towards the operators is lowered. From a neuroscientific standpoint, it is very clear that harsh language and rude manners generate annoyance, fear, and triggers the "fight or flight" response in our bodies. To avoid violent communication, observe what is happening (fact-checking), check the feelings of the other (and then yours), let the other express the need (and then express yours), and ask for a concrete and feasible request. All this is helped by the development of empathy, an intelligent one, not a naïve, sometimes useless sympathy; this is one of the most vital ways to avoid escalation into a tunnel of violence.

8.4.2 Reading the Narrative on Violence Written By a Doctor Who Prefers to Remain Anonymous

Definition of violence Treccani encyclopedia: "Act or behavior using physical force (with or without the use of weapons or other offensive means) to cause harm to others in person, property, or rights. In a broader sense, the abuse of force (also represented by words alone or by moral abuse, threats, blackmail) as a means of coercion oppression, i.e., to compel others to act or yield against their will."

"I am a psychiatrist now nearing retirement. In the last thirty years, I have spent in the company of the "insane" (those who, for common sense, are the dangerous, the violent), I have had countless physical encounters with them, but I have encountered violence maybe once or twice and in subjects who were delinquents. The insane, rather than attack defend themselves, theirs is not violence, but fear, and any of us would defend ourselves as we can if threatened, betrayed, and forced: this is their most common viewpoint. I only use the pronoun 'they' for brevity, but I want to point out that every encounter has been different, even the last one, last month, when a patient in the throes of a flare-up injured the tendon of a finger on my left hand. The orthopedists say that operating on it is not worth it and that the result could be worse than it is now. I look at my hand with that finger that doesn't stay up like before; it's constantly flexed and can't go straight anymore. I tell myself I'm not a pianist, and it's not that bad. That the prehensile strength is there after all and that, for me, it boils down to a question of aesthetics, but that's not true. My body is forever deformed, and I'll have to get used to it. I was almost fine for thirty years, but not this time; it could have been a lot worse, but that's not enough. The irreversibility of life events is the natural human condition, but the experience of this in one's flesh changes the extent of one's awareness forever.

My grandmother was a peasant woman, and when referring to someone who had an obvious physical impairment, she would say that the person had a leg, hand, or arm: 'offended', then, in pronouncing this word, she would lower her tone of voice and her gaze in a way that, in me as a child, commanded sacred respect. I, too, have an 'offended' finger that you can see, but I do not resent that patient: he was not violent at all; he was just terrified. What grieves me most about these years of work, now thirty-six, is far more violence, especially the invisible and unsuspected ones that are widespread at all levels in healthcare.

Health-related professions belong to those defined as ethical. Yet, human beings beyond their professional qualification cannot renounce the pleasure of imposing themselves on others and, in doing so, completely forget their mandate, or rather, find the most original compromises between this, their benefit, and the theoretical human respect on which ethics is based. Verbal violence is not always that of the frank insult; in some circles, phrases such as: 'He is good, but he does not obey (us)...' suffice. The violent insult is in the tone of the dots that follow, and it is far more effective than any profanity can contemplate; it is as devastating as a blow with the axe. "He does not obey"! Whoever utters this phrase at the right moment has 'forced the unfortunate one to surrender his or her will', knowing full well that this is what it takes for expediency to bring about what is reasonable to the one who is expedient regardless of any other value, principle or history. From this point onwards, the unfortunate 'is out of the game', and almost nothing can be done to him/her because he/she will have no power to reply. And here, the violence adds up simply and widely: the shift change does not come; it is delayed... they do not count. The news of the limited number of courses to attend always arrives out of time.

The news of the limited numbered course to attend always arrives out of time. The 'mangy' case always comes to him/her. If he/she has a problem, he/she keeps it. It can continue for years, but proving mobbing will still be difficult. The organization's manager fuels this climate because it serves the divide-and-conquer purpose, and imperceptible movements are enough to generate violence, which, however, must never be definitive because the scapegoat is indispensable anyway. Again, proving bossing is complicated. Alongside this is bureaucratic violence, one of the most despicable and insidious forms of prevarication and completely comparable to the invisible sniper who calmly aims, kills at a distance and disappears. Bureaucracy was originally supposed to be a guaranteed apparatus but, as Treccani reports: 'Weber spoke of an irreversible process of universal bureaucratization, which tended to imprison men in a web of minute rules and to subject them to the anonymous, irresponsible and ever more necessary power of bureaucratic apparatuses (...).

I remember a funny anecdote: one December a few years ago, I made a rejected holiday request because I had used up all my days for the year. I was astonished: I had practically only asked for summer holidays that year! I collected the attendance records for the previous months and found a series of randomly scattered and never-requested days off that heavily influenced the overall count. I asked the bureaucrat in charge about this, and he candidly replied that when he encountered an irregular stamping of the working day, he solved the problem by turning it into a holiday; for him, there was only the tripartite bureaucratic reality: either you work, or you are on sick leave or holiday: if they did not inform him of the sickness, it was a holiday for him! The fact that a failure to clock in could be due to a thousand factors (malfunctioning of the timekeeper, demagnetization of the card, loss, material or circumstantial impossibility, theft or whatever) did not interest him: according to him, allocating office leave was the most straightforward solution! Naturally, I informed him that I would immediately report him if he did not resolve the situation by the law. He did so but took great offence. This microscopic episode involving an official who is more naive and simpler than other colleagues have the merit of allowing, through its transparency, the substantial 'thought form' of the bureaucrat to be revealed. Colleagues far more skillful and cunning than our friend and, more or less in the service of this or that power, manage to cover up practices, block funds, jam up careers, increase waiting lists and so on, exercising daily violence with the utmost indifference. Bureaucracy is a very powerful machine; anyone with partial control over it can do a lot. Now, the Directors of the Health Authorities are appointed by the Regional Councils, administering from time to time based on the political consensus received, while the 'bureaucrats' are always the same.

There is violence by delegation, i.e., when another institution delegates to the health facilities out of supposed competence over the case.

This can happen without any forethought, without caring whether beds are available in a ward or not and what the presence of a prisoner in that ward entails. The police arrive with the prisoner proceed, and the violence involves everyone with an innocent lexicon: 'with planting was deemed necessary by the medical staff.' Who will be forced to do the planting? The nurse or the police? Whose responsibility is it for custody? Whose fault is it for care (if any)? Who is the prisoner: patient, dangerous offender or both?

More is needed; delegation may also concern those cases where it is established that a parent or parents are not fit to maintain parental authority for the most diverse reasons, and a child has to be entrusted to others.

The child is taken away from the family of origin, and in this context, psychiatric services are involved in managing the parents' reaction and 'I have seen things you humans could not imagine...' and it wasn't battleships on fire off the ramparts of Orion, it wasn't even a film.

There are, of course, much lower, and more obvious levels of violence. Harassment is a form of it that I have unfortunately encountered declined in many ways: by the established professional towards the young nurse or pretty patient; by the patient towards the doctor or nurse; by the patient blackmailing the professional with the lie of harassment from him and so on. All this creates impairments, mutilates, disarticulates, deforms, and distorts the soul and professionalism of the victims: it leaves them 'offended', irreversibly.

Continuing in the simplification of violence, one arrives at the use of physical force in actual beatings, and of these, among medical staff, I have no direct knowledge, but from others, I do.

Frequently in emergency rooms and by relatives of patients: it has happened to many and to me too, but it is becoming a ubiquitous phenomenon proportionally linked to the cultural and civil degradation that affects our country.

Finally, I would like to discuss an extreme form of violence: murder.

This also exists, and it recently happened to the psychiatrist colleague from Pisa, Barbara Capovani, who was bludgeoned to death by a 'patient/criminal': she had just left the hospital after a day's work one evening last April (2023). All Italian psychiatrists reacted with torchlight processions and demonstrations in every region of the country, spontaneous chats were formed with thousands of members, the Minister of Health showed his attention, and something was moving. But Barbara is dead, irreversibly dead, because this Collectivity, the Legislator, and the scientific interpretation of specific data has not yet decided where to draw the line between delinquency and madness, and this grey area that has persisted for decades suits many. In the meantime, Barbara is dead and not the only one but the last.

To conclude, I quote the term of reference for the following 'Code', Presidential Decree No 62 of April 16 2013 [1].

Regulation laying down a code of conduct for public employees, according to Article 54 of Legislative Decree No 165 of March 30 2001.

1. Published in the Official Journal No 129 of June 4 2013.

   Art. 1 General Provisions

1. This Code of Conduct, from now on referred to as the "Code," defines, for Article 54 of Legislative Decree No. 165 of March 302,001, the minimum duties of diligence, loyalty, impartiality and good conduct that civil servants are required to observe.

   Article 3 General principles

1. Employees shall observe the Constitution, serving the Nation with discipline and honour and conforming their conduct to the principles of good performance and impartiality of administrative action. The employee shall perform his/her duties by the law, pursuing the public interest without abusing his/her position or powers.

   It would be desirable to withstand all this violence until retirement, to get there with as minor offence as possible, assuming we get there...With discipline and honour."

   I am grateful for this wise and deep reflection about violence, grief for Barbara, an activist in Health Care, and sorrow and shame for the bureaucratic violence.

8.4.3 Learning What is Empathy from a Neuroscientific Point of View

Human empathy is the result of a biological summation between more primordial stages of the animal brain: the reptilian brain, or the limbic brain of mammals, including primates (when in danger, it prepares the body to either fight or flee, requires attachment and group recognition) and the telencephalon, developed in humans where cognitive comprehension areas are present [6]. These three parts are in constant interconnection with each other and are activated at different times depending on the environment. When the autonomic nervous system is continuously engaged in defensive activities, as can happen in traumatic situations or prolonged stress, it can become immensely challenging to foster empathic relationships, creating lasting damage to psycho-physical health status of an individual. Stephen Porges' Polyvagal Neuroscientific Theory has revealed that the parasympathetic system, functioning through the vagus nerve, is composed of two circuits belonging to different periods of our phylogenetic history. The ventrovagal one (more recent in phylogeny) drives the muscles of the face, voice and breathing. Meanwhile, the dorso-vagal one (older) maintains balance and control of basic visceral functions (stomach, small intestine, colon, bladder). In dangerous conditions, the former has a calming effect on the heart, reduces the sympathetic system's activation level and promotes social engagement behavior. In contrast, the older circuit has only one possible reaction: shutdown. Conversely, the sympathetic nervous system has an intermediate state responsible for responses in the event of danger from the attack/escape system.

It is not possible to ward off all dangers. Still, it is possible to create a safe space where the body—with its perception—feels at ease. The voice of the mother the first thing that the fetus perceives, and is, therefore, paramount to the development of the bond between mother and child (in fact, this may be the origin of the phrasing "mother tongue"). The human ear has evolved to extrapolate the sound of the human voice from background noise. It can distinguish whether the speaker is in danger or in a safe position based on the quality of the perceived voice. Low, sad sounds activate all the alarm systems in our body, while louder, more melodic sounds set the stage for tranquility. To create an empathic relationship, there must be a space of safety generated through voice, facial expressions, gaze, being seen and considered, and contact: now, during the Covid-era, contact, handshake, and embrace are all the more likely to be replaced by voice, a smile, and facial expression.

Also, from a neuroscientific point of view, the mirror neurons activated when an individual observes a purposeful action performed by another individual in our brain are an extraordinary discovery by Giacomo Rizzolatti for understanding the functioning of empathy. Specifically, when we see a person talking, we observe a bilateral activation of the brain's pre-motor system, which includes the language area, and thus, simply by listening, we are ready to respond; when we see a monkey, we observe in our brain, a bilateral pre-motor activation of reduced intensity; finally, when we hear a dog barking, there is a complete absence of motor reaction.

We know a dog is barking, but the human involvement is much lower than when a person speaks, predisposing humans to empathic sociality.

Affective empathy typically emerges in the second year of a child's life and is mainly dependent on the nature of human interactions; it is a function of caregiving style and family environment to support self-awareness and conscious concern for others, along with genetic factors.

In children with Asperger's syndrome, neuroimaging studies have shown that mirror neurons do not activate appropriately in response to external stimuli. When they speak, they are unfiltered or fail to read emotional signals. In fact, they struggle to understand other people's feelings through metaphorical language (they take words literally) and prefer solitude to relationships with others. Human contact is essential to communication for most human beings, but for people with the autistic spectrum, social relationships are experienced as a violation of their own space.

They are gifted with mathematical and logical intelligence, while empathy is the basis of intra- and interpersonal intelligence, as demonstrated by Howard Gardner. Lack of empathy is a trait of some personality disorders, such as narcissism or borderline disorder. Some neuroimaging studies show low brain activity in brain areas related to empathy in diagnosed narcissists.

In the end, empathy, whether emotional or cognitive, is the pillar to build relationships of trust that allow cooperation between individuals to overcome difficulties, build well-being and, in a historical sense, the evolution of humanity.

8.4.4 Mastering Style of Communication

Communication has three fundamental postures: passive, assertive, and aggressive. Passive behavior is accepting events or the actions of others without resistance. Some synonyms include submissive, yielding, obedient, meek, subdued, and deferential. It also means being weak and small.

Aggressive communication is "ready or likely to attack or confront," with synonyms including hostile, antagonistic, or belligerent. Shoulders become open, people stand up, the tune of voice shouts, and the person becomes big, filling the voids in the space.

Assertive is showing confidence and standing up for one's rights directly and honestly. Synonyms include self-confident, positive, self-assured, firm, and determined. Finding the right size of self-esteem within a group of colleagues, with a patient and his/her caregivers, with the health care management, and with the scientific community.

And now:

What is violence for you? How would you have been acting/reacting at the meeting with Dr. Kings of Hearts?

How would you act if you faced an angry colleague or patient at the threshold of verbal violence?

Would you like to write down two short narratives, one referring to a "violent" colleague or a "violent team" and a second one referring to "a violent" patient or a "violent caregiver"? Do you recall the facts? Were you passive, aggressive, or assertive? What are your feelings yet? Which could be your request now?

8.4.5 Finding Time to Say Hallo to Alice

Alice, Humpty Dumpty and the words in After the Looking Glass:

'I don't know what you mean by "glory,"' Alice said.
Humpty Dumpty smiled contemptuously. 'Of course, you don't—till I tell you. I meant, "There's a nice knock-down argument for you!"'
'But "glory" doesn't mean a nice knock-down argument,' Alice objected.
*"When I use a word," Humpty Dumpty said scornfully, **"it means just what I choose it to mean—neither more nor less."***
*"The question is," said Alice, **"whether you can make words mean so many different things."***
"The question is,"** said Humpty Dumpty, **"which is to be master—that's all."
*Alice was too puzzled to say anything, so Humpty Dumpty began again after a minute. "They have **a temper, some of them—particularly verbs; they're the proudest—adjectives you can do anything with, but not verbs**—however, I can manage the whole lot of them! Impenetrability! That's what I say!"*

"Would you tell me, please," said Alice *"what that means?"*
"Now you talk like a reasonable child," said Humpty Dumpty, *looking very pleased.*
'I meant by "impenetrability" that we've had enough of that subject, and it would be just as well if you'd mention what you mean to do next, as I suppose you don't mean to stop here all the rest of your life.'
"That's a great deal to make one word mean," Alice said thoughtfully.
"When I make a word do a lot of work like that," said Humpty Dumpty, *"I always pay it extra."*

Some subjects and people are impenetrable, and we get sick of always staying in the rabbit hole. The obscurity of some words and demands us to move forward, trying to escape an immovable situation. This is when Alice grows up and finds the courage to cross the looking mirror and see another face of reality: understanding the relationship she can have between her desires and the meanings of the words. Eventually, she learns to speak.

References

1. Bucknall V, Burwaiss S, MacDonald D, Charles K, Clement R. Mirror mirror on the ward, who's the most narcissistic of them all? Pathologic personality traits in health care. CMAJ. 2015;187(18):1359–63.
2. Neprash HT, et al. Association of primary care visit length with potentially inappropriate prescribing. JAMA Health Forum. 2003;4(3):e230052.
3. Tai-Seale M, et al. Time allocation in primary care office visits. Health Serv Res. 2007;42(5):1871–94.
4. Pitts E, Schaller DJ. Violent patients. National Institute for Health; 2022.
5. Civilotti C, Berlanda S, Iozzino L. Hospital-Based Healthcare Workers Victims of Workplace Violence in Italy: A Scoping Review, Cristina Civilotti, Sabrina Berlanda, Laura Iozzino. Int J Environ Res Public Health. 2021;18(11):5860.
6. Marini MG. Treccani. Le parole del XXI secolo. s.d.

Chapter 9
The Ceaseless Cycle of Violence, Cause of Malaise and Cooperation of Human Beings as Cause of Well Being

Our contemporary age is a period in which human beings, with incredible acceleration, have produced (and are continually bringing about) a technological revolution that has had a frightening impact. What do I mean when I say "frightening?" Let us review some statistics; 10% of the total population on earth holds 75% of the global wealth, we have a population that is very difficult to feed and provide healthcare and hospitality to. Today there are about eight billion inhabitants on earth, as of November 2022, compared to the people of one and seven billion estimated in 1910. Moreover, we cannot fail to mention the damage, most likely irreversible, done to our planet that have led to global warming and thus, the desertification and inability to cultivate food [1].

9.1 The Historical Era of the Anthropocene

Anthropos, "at the center," not as the crossroads of art and science, as seen in humanism, but in the worst sense with a social system that destroys the planet and creates inequities in the distribution of wealth. The "magnificent progressive fortunes," caustically described by the Italian poet Giacomo Leopardi counteracted by the Machiavellian limitation *'Ipse faber fortune suae,'* or "each is the maker of his fortune." The drastic successes and well-being of a few, that have led to painfully gradual improvements in the standard of living of the many seem to no longer nullify the dissatisfaction of the multitude. We can say that neuroscientist Iain Mc Gil-Christ is sadly correct when he states that we are slaves to the left hemisphere of the brain; we wish it could be solely a center of logic and rationality; instead, it come with the cost of greed and short-term vision [2]. Having we betrayed our right hemisphere, the one of humanism, art and science as intuition, and empathy with others? It would seem so, that we have left humanities and humanism by the large, and it is made apparent by the same method of statistical analysis that we prize as a society, that has revealed demographic disparities in well-being and malaise ([3] as in Fig. 9.1).

Parallel to the evolution of scientific and technological discoveries, Sigmund Freud, at the beginning of the last century, hypothesizes, based on empirical cases, how our mind is made and discovers its "monstrous side," not so much identified in the Es (the pleasure principle that brings us back to the lost state of nature) but in the loss of the reality principle, the Ego, and especially in the Superego. It is the Superego that creates the disturbed, neurotic, and dare I say, degenerating human being. The physician Sigmund Freud operated in Vienna in the late 1800s and early 1900s in a very restrictive environment, determined by subterranean forces, such as those that governed sexuality. He had a fascination with the things that individuals hid in the closet of their minds. I would say remove the white and golden Habsburg stucco, along with the many inner conflicts, the many faces of the human being. Next, to the joy of life of the Es, Freud with the Superego, in his masterful book, *Civilization and its Discontents* [4], gives in advance an explanation of what generally happens in hyper-hierarchical civilizations, where people's faculty of thought is taken away. For example, it will be precisely that hypertrophic. Over redundant Superego who will "trivially"-I borrow Hannah Arendt's title, "The Banality of Evil" [5] execute the orders to send six million Jews to gas chambers, as reported by Nazi hierarchs in the Nuremberg trial. *"We were carrying out the orders,"* and Arendt comments with dismay, *"How is it possible that they did not think? Didn't they ask themselves ethical questions?"* and the hierarchs replied, "An order is an order." I need to specify that in these lines, I'm assigning to "superego" the despotic meaning, and not a moralizing sense.

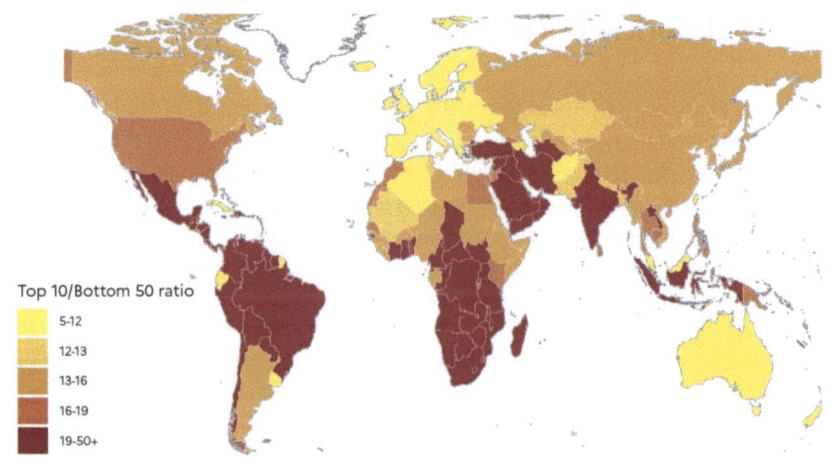

Interpretation: In Brazil, the bottom 50% earns 29 times less than the top 10%. The value is 7 in France. Income is measured after pension and unemployment payments and benefits received by individuals but before other taxes they pay and transfers they receive.
Source and series: wir2022.wid.world/methodology.

Fig. 9.1 Distribution of world income levels

9.1 The Historical Era of the Anthropocene

And it is the Superego of the norm, even the most terrible one, internalized to the point where guilt for what has been accomplished disappears. The ethics of the reality principle, "compassion," "Humanitas" burned away by that totalitarianism and the other totalitarian regimes of the twentieth century.

While through vaccinations, the potabilization of water, the discovery of antibiotics, created wealth and extended life in some countries, genocides and massacres were committed in others. We cannot forget the Armenians in 1912, the "Great Leap Forward" campaign promoted by Mao between 1949 and 1976 that resulted in the deaths of 40 million dead Chinese, the Holodomor (1932–1933) caused by Stalin in Ukraine, who then with his gulags and deportations suppressed some 30 million people; the futility of Vietnam, the wars in the Middle East, the Desaparecidos in Argentina and Chile, the Hutus and Tutsis in Rwanda, and the genocide of the Serbs in Milosevic's mass graves. Now we are facing another war, this time almost at home, between Russia and Ukraine.

Not only are technologies to better health and well-being improving, but also technologies to cause death and destruction. And so, it was Freud who, though at the beginning of his studies contemplated only the pleasure instinct, after World War I, added an instinct previously unpronounceable to humankind: the death instinct.

Alongside this, *homo*, as Marcuse declared, is kept controlled only through consumption, hence the *One-Dimensional Man* [6] is born, taking far more than he gives to the planet. Enlightening and prescient is Italo Calvino short novel, *Invisible Cities*, written in 1972 [7] about the city of Leonia, that continues every day to consume to a bitter end. I see much in this short tale of the contemporary condition of some affluent countries that then go and export their garbage outside, to other regions, because they do not know where or what to do with it.

Here is a brief excerpt from *Invisible Cities* to contemplate on:

> The city of Leonia remakes itself every day: every morning, the population wakes up amidst crisp sheets, washes with soapsuds freshly peeled from their wrappers, wears shiny new robes, pulls out tin cans still intact from the most perfected refrigerator, listens to the latest nursery rhymes from the most recent model of appliance. On the sidewalks, wrapped in terse plastic bags, the remains of yesterday's Leonia await the garbage wagon. Not only the crushed tubes of toothpaste, electrocuted light bulbs, newspapers, containers, and packaging materials, but also water heaters, encyclopedias, pianos, and porcelain services: rather than by the things of every day are manufactured and sold bought, the opulence of Leonia is measured by the things that are thrown away every day to make way for new ones. So much so that one wonders if Leonia's true passion is, as they say, to enjoy new and different things, or not rather to expel, to remove from oneself, to cleanse oneself of a recurring impurity. What is certain is that garbage collectors are welcomed as angels, and their task of eliminating the re-statements of yesterday's existence is surrounded by silent respect, like a ritual that inspires devotion, or maybe just because once the stuff is thrown away, no one wants to have to think about it anymore. Where the garbage collectors take their load every day, no one wanders outside the city, sure, but every year, the city expands, and the garbage collectors have to stop farther away; the impressiveness of the throwaway increases, and the piles rise, stratify, unfold over a wider perimeter.
>
> Add that the more Leonia's art excels at fabricating new materials, the more the garbage improves its substance to withstand time, weather, fermentation and combustion. It is a fortress of indestructible remnants that surrounds Leonia, towering over it like an acrochorus of mountains. The result is this: the more Leonia expels stuff, the more it accumu-

lates; the scales of its past are welded into an armor that cannot be removed and repairs itself every day; the city retains all of itself in the only definitive form: that of yesterday's garbage piling up on the garbage of the other day and years and lustres. Little by little, Leonia's garbage would invade the world if the endless garbage heap were not pressing; beyond the extreme ridge were garbage heaps from other cities, repelling the mountains of garbage away from themselves. Perhaps the whole world beyond Leonia's borders is covered with craters of garbage, each with an uninterruptedly erupting metropolis at its centre. The borders between foreign and enemy cities are infected ramparts where the debris of one and the other propped up each other, overlapping and mingling. The more their height grows, the more the danger of the landslides looms: all it takes is for a tin can, an old tire, a splintered flask to roll on Leonia's side and an avalanche of mismatched shoes, calendars of years gone by, dried flowers will submerge the city in its past that it vainly tried to repel, mixed with that of the other neighboring cities, finally clean. A cataclysm will level the sordid mountain range, erase all traces of the metropolis always dressed up. Already from the neighboring cities, they are ready with steam rollers to level the ground, extend into the new territory, enlarge themselves, drive away the new filth.

"Slow violence," a term coined by Bob Nixon in 2011 [8], describes harmful human behaviors towards earth; this violence occurs gradually and is not necessarily visible. Slow violence is "incremental and accretive;" its key outcomes are environmental degradation, long-term pollution and climate change. Slow violence is also closely linked to many instances of environmental racism. Environmental racism and ecological racism are forms of institutional racism leading to landfills, incinerators, and hazardous waste disposal being disproportionately placed in BIPOC communities. Internationally, it is also associated with extractivism, which sets the environmental burdens of mining, oil extraction, and industrial agriculture upon indigenous peoples and poorer nations inhabited mainly by people of color. Bob Nixon states that people lacking resources or living in poverty are the main casualties of slow violence, as it is "built on the bedrock of social inequality." People who must migrate because of mega-dam construction, massive deforestation, or land exploitation for drilling will never have the legal status of before. They are not even nomads; since they were not born as nomads, they become rootless. These people who had to quite their homeland manage their life in a "picturesque" easy, trying to survive daily. Almost two-thirds of the planet suffers from this "slow violence" illness that pollutes our ecosystem.

From an epidemiological point of view, the climate change of the Anthropocene age might cause, according to the forecast of the WHO, the following outcomes: higher temperatures, rising sea levels, and flooding affect all aspects of food and nutrition security. Furthermore climate-related reductions in agricultural and marine productivity, biodiversity loss, volatility in food prices and disruptions in food imports further affect the quality, quantity and diversity of food consumed, leading to further food and nutrition crises. Changing temperature and precipitation patterns also increase the suitability of conditions for transmitting mosquito-borne, tick-borne and rodent-borne diseases in many regions. If prevention methods are not strengthened, this could increase the over 700,000 deaths from vector-borne diseases yearly.

Acute mental health conditions such as anxiety, depression and post-traumatic stress can be experienced following extreme weather events. The cumulative effect of loss of livelihood, displacement, disrupted social cohesion and uncertainty from climate change can also result in longer-term mental health disorders, adding to the already enormous global challenges in mental health. Estimating the entire health burden of climate change is challenging. However, the assessment is established by looking at a small subset of causal pathways [9].

The one-dimensional man, the homo inhabitant of Leonia, who is making the earth an immense rubbish bin, changing its climate by polluting it, subjecting it to plutocracy and consumption, is a representation of the "Western" Superego: hyper well-being, consumption at all costs, or following the current locution, the "wow effect," which burns overnight in the subjectivity of the human being, but impacts, almost irreversibly, our planet. Unfortunately, there are proofs for assigning most of these responsibilities to the WASP, White Anglo-Saxon Protestant Men. Indeed, there is a cultural effect and a gender effect. Men drill oil, and women are involved in the caring profession.

Yet, slow violence has its diametrically opposite vector coexisting with the continuing demand for freedom (not liberalism), democracy, self-expression, and self-creation, explained in the most significant human rights ever being written outside a utopian novel right into the twentieth century.

9.1.1 What Health, What Rights?

After World War II, people who had survived the horrors of both wars had hoped to change the course of events, and they succeeded in part. In 1948, the year of the greatest ideals, the World Health Organization, founded precisely to deal with the Spanish flu pandemic in 1918, defined health as the absence of disease and the complete physical, psychological and social well-being. Here, we understand that it is impossible to separate health from well-being, they are synonymous. So, it is not enough to "save oneself," to "survive," in health from the Latin word *salvus*, which means "safe," for WHO health means "to exist well." The fourth dimension, existential and spiritual well-being, has been added to the three bio-psycho and socio dimensions in the last forty years [10].

Not everyone in WHO agrees on adding spirituality to well-being since, for many scholars, this arises from the intertwining of the previous three dimensions. However, we feel we include it as an item because it is a treasure chest of values and attitudes that a person or a group of people possess that do not necessarily fall back on or derive from revealed religions. This may lead us to look for values even in the ancient traditions of the past that might have had their meaning taken from as much as it has been given form the ecosystem. The characters of the homo faber and one-dimensional man stopped doing, took and are taking far more from the ecosystem: and now maybe it's too late, to nourish our planet and our soul.

9.2 Human Rights

In 1948, the Charter of Human Rights was born, of which we quote the thirty Articles signed by the United Nations:

Article 1: All humans are born free and equal in dignity and rights. They are endowed with reason and conscience and must act toward one another in a spirit of brotherhood.

Article 2: Everyone is entitled to all the rights and freedoms outlined in this Declaration, without distinction of any kind, whether because of race, color, sex, language, religion, political or other opinion, national or social origin, wealth, birth, or other status. No distinction shall also be established based on the political, legal or international status of the country or territory to which a person belongs, whether independent, under trusteeship or non-self-governing, or subject to any limitation of sovereignty.

Article 3: Everyone has the right to life, liberty, and security of his or her person.

Article 4: No individual shall be held in a state of slavery or servitude; slavery and the slave trade shall be prohibited in any form.

Article 5: No individual shall be subjected to torture or cruel, inhuman or degrading treatment or punishment.

Article 6 Everyone has the right everywhere to the recognition of his or her legal personality.

Article 7: Everyone is equal before the law and is entitled, without discrimination, to equal protection by the law. All are entitled to equal protection against any discrimination in violation of this Declaration as against any incitement to such discrimination.

Article 8: Everyone shall have the right to an effective remedy before competent courts of law acts that violate the fundamental rights granted by the constitution or law.

Article 9: No individual shall be arbitrarily arrested, detained or exiled.

Article 10: Everyone shall have the right, in a position of complete equality, to a fair and public hearing before an independent and impartial tribunal for the determination of his or her rights and duties, as well as of the merits of any criminal charge against him or her.

Article 11 1. Every individual accused of a crime shall be presumed innocent until his guilt has been legally proven in a public trial in which he has had all the guarantees necessary for his defense. No individual shall be convicted of any commission or omission that did not constitute a crime under domestic or international law at the time it was perpetrated. Similarly, no supra-judicial punishment shall be imposed than applicable when the crime was committed.

Article 12: No individual shall be subjected to arbitrary interference with his private life, family, home, correspondence, or injury to his honor and reputation. Everyone has the right to be legally protected against such interference or damage.

Article 13 1. Everyone has the right to freedom of movement and residence within the borders of each state. 2. Everyone has the right to leave any country, including his own, and return to his country.

Article 14 1. Everyone has the right to seek and enjoy in other countries asylum from persecution. 2. This right shall not be invoked if the individual is wanted for non-political crimes or actions contrary to the purposes and principles of the United Nations.

Article 15 1. Everyone has the right to a nationality. No individual shall be arbitrarily deprived of his or her citizenship nor of the right to change citizenship.

Article 16 1. Men and women of suitable age can marry and find a family without race, citizenship, or religion limitations. They shall have equal rights about marriage, during and upon its dissolution. 2. Marriage may be concluded only with the free and full consent of the prospective spouses. 3. The family is society's natural and fundamental nucleus and has the right to be protected by society and the state.

Article 17 1. Everyone has the right to have property of his own or in common with others. No individual shall be arbitrarily deprived of his property.

Article 18: Everyone has the right to freedom of thought, conscience, and religion; this right includes the freedom to change one's religion or belief and the freedom to manifest, either alone or in common, and whether in public or in private, one's religion or belief in teaching, practice, worship, and observance of rites.

Article 19: Everyone has the right to freedom of opinion and expression, including the right not to be harassed for his or her opinion and to seek, receive and disseminate information and ideas through any medium and without regard to frontiers.

Article 20 1. Everyone has the right to freedom of peaceful assembly and association. No one shall be compelled to join an association.

Article 21 1. Everyone has the right to participate in the government of his or her country, directly or through freely chosen representatives. 2. Everyone has the right to equal access to public employment in his or her country. 3. The people's will be the basis of the government's authority; this will shall be expressed through periodic and genuine elections, effected by universal and equal suffrage, secret ballot, or an equivalent procedure of liberation.

Article 22 Everyone, as a member of society, has the right to social security, as well as to the realization through national effort and international cooperation about the organization and resources of each state of the economic, social, and cultural rights indispensable to his dignity and the free development of his personality.

Article 23 1. Everyone has the right to work, free choice of employment, just and satisfactory working conditions and protection against unemployment. 2. Everyone, without discrimination, has the right to equal pay for equal work. 3. Everyone who works has the right to just and satisfactory remuneration that ensures for himself and his family an existence in conformity with human dignity and supplemented, if necessary, by other means of social protection. 4. Everyone can establish trade unions and join them to defend their interests.

Article 24: Everyone has the right to rest and recreation, including a reasonable limitation of working hours and periodic paid vacations.

Article 25: Everyone has the right to a standard of living sufficient to ensure the health and well-being of himself and his family regarding food, clothing, housing, and necessary medical care and social services. He has the right to security in case of unemployment, sickness, disability, widowhood, old age, or other loss of livelihood due to circumstances beyond his control. Motherhood and childhood are entitled to special care and assistance. All children shall enjoy the same social protection, whether born in or out of marriage.

Article 26 1. Everyone has the right to education. Education must be free, at least as far as the elementary and fundamental classes are concerned. Elementary education must be compulsory. Technical and vocational education must be available to all, and higher education must be equally accessible based on merit. 2. Education must be directed toward fully developing human personality and strengthening respect for human rights and fundamental freedoms. It shall promote understanding, tolerance, and friendship among all nations, racial and religious groups and further the work of the United Nations in maintaining peace. 3. Parents have the right of priority in choosing the kind of education to give their children.

Article 27 1. Everyone has the right to participate in the community's cultural life, enjoy the arts and participate in scientific progress and its benefits. 2. Every individual has the right to protect the moral and material interests resulting from any scientific, literary, and artistic production of which he or she is the author.

Article 28: Everyone has the right to a social and international order in which the rights and liberties outlined in this Declaration can be fully recognized.

Article 29 1. Everyone has duties to society, in which alone the free and full development of his personality is possible. 2. In the exercise of his rights and freedoms, each person shall be subject only to such limitations as are prescribed by law to ensure the re-recognition and respect for the rights and freedoms of others and to meet the just requirements of morality, public order, and the general welfare in a democratic society. 3. These rights and freedoms may in no case be exercised contrary to the purposes and principles of the United Nations.

Article 30 Nothing in this Declaration may be interpreted as implying a right to any State, group or person to engage in any activity or perform any act aimed at destroying any of the rights and freedoms set forth herein.

Without wanting to make equations of which rights belong to which field, security, freedom, recognition, health, welfare, and try another exercise: how many of these statements do we still feel are valid? And how much have we carried out? One only must look at the FAO [11] report to read that in 2021, there were 812 million people in the world suffering from severe malnutrition, most of them children and most of them in Africa, consistent with the trend in the distribution of money, that divide in which wealth continuously accumulates in fewer hands. And again, detentions for different political beliefs and torture happen, albeit rarely, even in our European countries. Let us count the femicides, of which Italy has the darkest flag in Europe.

9.2 Human Rights

And slavery, has it been eliminated? Slavery was never actually abolished. Instead, it has redefined itself into newer forms [12]. One of its manifestations is in the form of worker exploitation. Capitalism has led to severe exploitation of workers working in the factories, where they are forced to work for long hours in extremely harsh conditions to make a living to serve the luxuries of the rich-income class. Indeed, they are almost working as slaves, and this in most countries, with a causal effect relationship between wealth and health.

Although the entitlement narrative is epic, history has indicated the coexistence of good and evil in human beings, as described by Yuval Harari in his brief history of the Sapiens: [13] "The animal that became a god... we have dominated our environment, increased food production, co-built cities, founded empires and created distant trade networks. But have we decreased the amount of suffering in the world? Time and again, massive increases in human power have not necessarily improved the well-being of individual Sapiens and have usually caused immense suffering to other animals." While imagine falls into Freudian ES, the Utopic "locus mundi," historian Harari removes the veil from our eyes and gives us a sense of reality.

On the other hand, if we look at the studied history, amid old types of slavery, serfdom and inhumane working conditions, we can hope to have made progress on paper. We may find utopians in a dystopian world with islands of balanced reality. For people with disabilities, we know how much more stigma there was; they were sometimes suppressed from an early age and without any feeling of guilt. The Homo Faber, "The Man Who Makes," serves as a profound metaphor for the person who is unable to "produce sustenance and wealth" as an error of nature. Or a terrible chastisement of God, sanctioning discrimination for the person and the family. A scarlet letter that can persist for generations.

Pause reader...

Maybe you are a student who wishes to become an excellent medical doctor, or perhaps you are a nurse or a policy maker for healthcare services. Why all these statements about historical and legal frameworks? Because we must know them before and as we are looking after and caring for both ourselves and others. I am confident you can find the technical features of running the correct diagnosis during your internship and, maybe, with good technology. In this metaverse, you can practice yourself doing surgery on virtual patients. But this competence, of becoming more and more competent in Human skills (rights, empathy, compassion) and being aware of human limits (tyranny, brutality, violence), must be a persistent tension in our professional and personal lives. Otherwise, and this is a lively potential threat, AI like Chat GPT could wipe all of us out.

What we can do with these rights is analyze the communication style of language. The first thing we may notice is the abundance of universalism, sounds polite and professional, but also with a drive towards "generalizations." Words and phrases such as, "all," "everyone," "equality," "men and women," "rights," and "duties" aim at universality. There seems to be more rights than duties.

The communication style on the XX right is Epic and Religious, very much recalling the Law of Moses or the Quran, put in an imperative tense, with no other options available. They are written as a truism, but they, unfortunately, create significant fictions, also covered by ideology and not only ideals, which do not consider the complexity of the human being in all his/her shades from white to black.

Since these goals are so far away to reach, this communication genre tends to create a false perception of reality. Again, a mature Ego is lacking in his/her adult phase. I'm not against these principles, but I find this way of communication ineffective, naïve, and aggressive, lacking criticism and failing to acknowledge that we are still animals, passionate about achieving. And that we are also individuals, not only a herd of people.

Take the first article, 1: "All human beings are born free and equal in dignity and rights. They are endowed with reason and conscience and must act toward one another in a spirit of brotherhood. "Aggressive and stiff communication style: why should one feel to be a brother to someone who invaded his/her land?

What about changing this dogma in this possibility to improve? "Human beings are born free and equal in dignity and rights, with diversity in intelligences, emotions, and consciousness. They can act toward one another in a spirit of brotherhood and sisterhood"—assertive and open communication style, including diversities and potential.

9.3 Rights for Disabled People

Rights for disabled people moved and moved slowly. It was not until 1975 that the term "Disabled" appeared in the UN Declaration, replacing "handicapped." In this period, disability strictly concerns the subject's health, i.e., the approach to disability is a health one. It is this language that represents one of the significant limitations of this view, namely that everything must be consequential:

- first, the impairment, understood as a physical or psychological anomaly,
- then possibly the disability, conceived as inaptitude to a model,
- and finally, the probable disadvantage of society, defined as a handicap.

It was only in 2001 that the ICF (International Classification of Functioning, Disability and Health) [14] and the World Health Organization turned over a new leaf, adopting a new approach, i.e., from the medical model to the bio-psycho-social model. By shifting the focus from the reductive view of disability as merely linked to physical or mental impairment to the needs of the person's environment—the social, cultural, economic, physical, and technological environment—"Disability" has thus come to mean "an unfavorable relationship between a person and his or her health condition and environment." Therefore, if we follow the logic of this new definition, "any person at any time of life may have a health condition which in an unfavorable context becomes a disability." Between disability, fragility, and vulnerability, the step is tiny.

The UN Convention on the Rights of Persons with Disabilities of 2006 (in Italy Law 18/09) states that, "Disability is the result of the interaction between persons

9.3 Rights for Disabled People

with impairments and behavioral and environmental barriers, which impede their full and effective participation in society on an equal basis with others."

In the UN Convention, these are the principal rights that affect an estimated one billion disabled people on earth. The principle of "reasonable accommodation" (which means creating necessary and appropriate modifications and adjustments that do not impose a disproportionate or undue burden, where necessary in a specific case, to ensure that persons with disabilities enjoy or exercise on an equal basis with others all human rights and fundamental freedoms). The principle encompasses all of the following dimensions:

- Non-discrimination (children, adults and older people, women and men)
- Accessibility (the removal of architectural barriers)
- Situations of risk and humanitarian emergency
- Equal recognition before the law
- Access to justice
- Freedom from violence and exploitation
- Protection of the person's physical and mental integrity
- Respect for home and family
- Education
- Health
- Habilitation and rehabilitation
- Adequate living standards and social protection (social services must come into play in cases of disability: the family cannot be left alone)
- Political participation

These are beautiful declarations, yet there are so many gaps in their implementation. If the health part is still partly covered by the medical care service (and fortunately in most European countries free of charge), the remaining claims, including social services, which should also take care of integration into the world of work—the first point "accommodation"—are often disconnected from healthcare and are still linked to the religious and not for profit organizations. Although the importance of the third sector is fundamental, we understand that we are using "charitable and humanitarian'" organizations, and not applying our rights through the enactment of laws. Caring for someone living with a disability in such a way that honors the four dimensions (biological, psychological, social and spiritual) is not a universally applied right but becomes, in some lands, near and far, a humanitarian, voluntaristic and occasional act. However, if we go back in history from the disabled children "killed" because they are non-disabled in Roman society, or the disability seen as a divine condemnation and guilt to be atoned for, we have certainly made progress.

Examining the communication style, we made some progress also, compared to the language used in 1948 for human rights. I find very sensible that the principle of "reasonable accommodation" implies that everyone has to be taken care of, but according to the specific need and the specific culture of any particular context. While the principles of 1948 were absolute rights, today, rights are pondered for what is at stake. There is understandable tension, communication is full of potential, and ethics is more than a simple moralistic genre.

Therefore, it is tough to apply these values. There are biological explanations like Merleau Ponty's observation of a phenomenon in which we tend to avoid Physical Disability out of an instinct of self-preservation. We realize that from a physiological point of view, the inclusion of disability is not such a "spontaneous" phenomenon but an achievement; people must be educated since they are children to the inclusion of disability. Our "lizard brain," has within it a part that calls for its survival first," and if there is something "altered" ("not similar") in the other it tends, without an educational pathway to the civilization of accompaniment, to retreat, leaving "the diverse" lonely, isolated, and discriminated against [15]. Yet we can learn so many extraordinary lessons from those with a disability, particularly how to read reality with a unique set of eyes.

Despite understanding the reason why, we react this way towards those with disabilities, the human being in the contemporary age is backward. Even though care and health technologies are progressing vertiginously, there is a lack of cross-fertilization between knowledge, like a tower of Babel in which social services do not communicate enough with doctors, doctors with teachers, and employers do not understand their employees. In some cases, companies, despite the local laws, do not want to hire people from "protected categories." Although Italy, I repeat it, has many laws to protect workers, its application often leaves something to be desired, and private, especially small size, companies tend to pay the fee for not hiring disabled people, after a very short-sighted cost benefit analysis, instead of going for the inclusion process of people with mental and physical disabilities. What looks normal is privileged in our working society, despite the United Nations rules.

At ISTUD with LICE, *Lega contro l'Epilessia* (League against the Epilepsy), we have collected narratives of people living with epilepsy, which in some forms can be defined as a disability. Here are some written anonymous witnesses.

Narrative of a man, 40 years old, with epilepsy on his job expectations and experience

> *I studied at the University of Catania, at the same university in Rome, and obtained a Ph.D. In the meantime, I was undergoing treatment at Meyer Hospital in Florence.*
>
> *We "discovered" with my family in 1996 after moving from a small town to Catania; I don't remember having any manifestations at school. During my school years, I consulted professionals on the subject to understand what my epilepsy was derived from, both in Sicily and Rome. The seizures evolved and became more intense during university.*
>
> *I most enjoyed helping others and teaching; my experiences led me to become a social worker with many difficulties dictated by the constant therapy changes and trips to Florence (at Meyer). At first, of course, I had no limitations. I went out with my friends, studied with some difficulty, and drove. Workwise, I've always liked teaching and dealing with others, even through voluntary work. I had some psychological limitations when I had my first convulsive attacks.*
>
> *I wanted to become a university professor and a professor of human rights, this I could not do for reasons of treatment when it was discovered that I had "limitations" (for example, when I had manifestations of my pathology in the classroom or when I started to stop driving).*
>
> *People close to me have always helped me. I attended as a volunteer, as the manager is an oratory and does not always understand. Fundamental has been my family, cousins,*

9.3 Rights for Disabled People

sister, and brother-in-law. Some of my colleagues, and now my wife. Also, my therapist friend helped me get unstuck in some things.

My employers don't know what kind of pathology I have. They know I can't drive any more, but they don't do anything to help me, considering that I work in a different city from where I stay.

The beginning of the job search was necessary. I was still driving; pharmacologically, the pathology was controlled. I did various jobs, but I had to leave some for various reasons, even though they gave me a lot of incentives. The job interviews all went well, although with a bit of insecurity; more than job interviews, I did competitions until last year, where I found a job that could be permanent, but which made me travel a lot by car; it was not possible to get there by public transport. Two years ago, I had a bad accident because I had a crisis in the car and stopped driving ultimately.

The first experiences at work went well, but as I said, I was stressed, which increased the crisis. Until two years ago, my relationship with my neighbor, as a social worker, was very stressful and by no means did it improve my auras. I used to get up early in the morning and return very late.

The treatment of epilepsy from 96 to today has significantly changed because the drugs and therapy have changed. In addition, I used a professional psychotherapist for a while to help me accept and cope with the moment of crisis. The most challenging and most frustrating moment was my treatment at Meyer. To date, I have found epileptologists here in Sicily who are helping me a lot in the direction of treatment.

In the beginning, I still didn't understand it well, even though my sister, for a time, suffered from epilepsy, a minor illness which gradually ended at the age of eighteen. I felt myself getting more and more confused and more and more frightened as I went along.

As I went on, I began to cope better, though always with difficulty, also because there were periods when I had a few chronic tonic seizures. Several times, however, I ended up in hospital. Fortunately, at work and university, I had no manifestations also dictated by the positive stress it induced in me.

Today, my crises are more present; above all, they manifest themselves in hours that would be difficult to explain here. Today, I have given up many things: a job that could be stable, moving freely by car, and staying alone at home with my father, who unfortunately suffers from Parkinson's. I work when my colleague goes to work as I take the train, and then this colleague accompanies me to an appointment, but I always have faith now I am in my forties. I believe in medicine, although sometimes the sense of frustration returns.

I have become more mature and nearly more aware; I go to the gym, where my trainer knows about my pathology. I do not have children for fear, perhaps in the past, of being unable to care for them myself when my wife is not at home but at work.

The experience of the pandemic changed me at times. It knocked me down two months before I had VNS (Vagus Nerve Stimulation) implanted. And during the pandemic, I had various tonic and chronic crises. I reacted well to the pandemic, albeit like everyone else, with much stress, but mainly because of my serene and accepting character, even after my experiences.

I like my work, especially in healthcare. I keep going when I cannot be helped by my employers, as I said, but by my colleagues, some of them help me and advise me. I have some regrets. I would have liked to work for human rights since I also have a master's degree taken with so much effort. But fatigue and events did not make me continue that path. Today my job is more and more stressful, mainly because of travelling. And if I told my employers that I had the pathology, I am sure they would let me down since I am, unfortunately, on a freelance contract.

I tried to get in us a support teacher, but unfortunately, nothing.

Relations are very good with my colleagues; some know about the pathology, and some know about the operation, but my employer, I repeat it, does not know anything even though I work in a Rehabilitation centre; too ignorance(?) since I have asked several times to be *approached in Catania. Unfortunately, I can only do it in my presence because right now, I would need to work remotely, given the great difficulty in public transport, to move from one province to another and get paid after three degrees. I don't visit the occupational doctor since I am a freelancer.*

There are no associations near me for those who suffer from this pathology. I refer to the LICE, who helps me a lot when I have questions; my neurologist also helps me and is always available. My family is always there for me, even though my elderly parents, especially my mother, don't know many things to avoid stressing them out. My wife is a great reference point, although I try not to stress her too much. Another significant reference point is my sister.

I tried to get in as a support teacher, but unfortunately, the treatment of epilepsy is long, difficult and always changing. The luck is that here in Catania, there are great professionals who, first of all, understand the patient, listen to and don't judge...By now, I am almost very organized as I always walk with epilepsy drugs, and a magnet is watching for the moment I fall; I warn my Caregivers.

Tomorrow, I don't know. I'm a bit discouraged, mainly because, at present, I only work once a week because working in another municipality would stress me too much. I need to be at home with someone anyway. I would like to be understood; I would like there to be no prejudice; I would like it to be talked about more; I would like employers to understand people with my pathology more, and I would not want to get tired of my job even though it is too late.

Maybe I would like to go back to university.

Writing my story has, above all, made me reflect. There are so many things I would have liked to write about. Still, I have, fortunately or unfortunately, forgotten over time, but when they come to my mind, I don't know how to deal with them. Sometimes, they have, as my therapist told me, made me more ready to help others and more prepared to listen, but with so many frailties, I always thank my family, and I thank my wife.

Narrative of a woman with epilepsy, aged 40, from Liguria, and her experience with work

I graduated in Public Relations and Advertising. In the meantime, I suffered from anorexia nervosa and spent a year in a centre specializing in eating disorders. I fell ill with anorexia because ever since I fell ill with epilepsy at 13, I was always told not to tell anyone about it so as not to be discriminated against. Still, it was a huge burden to keep inside. Despite this, after graduating, I immediately got a job with a lot of responsibility, first as a trainee and then as an events manager in a large structure. Formatively, it was very nice, but it was very stressful. I had no timetable and was often on the road at trade fairs and always on call. It was not the best for my health, and it suffered. I quit my job and did some part-time work (clothing manager for a chain of shops, call centre...) meanwhile I resumed my studies. I was called to work on a fashion project at a prestigious university. I oversaw cataloguing, researching and selecting the material to be included in the project with a small team I was coordinating. The work was healthier in pace and hours but more repetitive. When the project was finished, I won a scholarship for a window dressing and visual merchandising course, qualifying with flying colors.

In the meantime, my epilepsy got worse. I could no longer do things as I had earlier, and I had to change treatment several times because I was always sick—the most harmful period of my life. I was humiliated. I used to perform well, though I could barely do everyday things. I didn't show up for interviews anymore and didn't know what to say or how I would be. It felt like a nightmare. I fell back on occasional collaborations in a showroom with numerous stop-offs, and then I enrolled in a Chinese course at the Italian Chinese consulate. It was tough mentally to be lucid at times, and I was terrified of having seizures in class, but I managed to get to level 3 with exams and certifications. Despite my numerous setbacks over the last few years, I never gave up. I took a certification in image counselling, took a few courses, and did some counselling. I worked freelance, organizing small events for shops and individuals. I realized that my health is important, and I want to protect it. I worked for a car magazine, did marketing and was a columnist in the lifestyle section. Currently, I am setting up on my own to do events, communication, and image consultancy. I seek a good compromise between my health, work skills, and resourcefulness.

I was very good at school. Nobody ever knew about my problems, not even the teachers. This created a lot of stress for me because I often had check-ups to do or spent days in hospitals. I was hospitalized several times. The situation also made me very uncomfortable with classmates to whom I did not know what to say. I often had to make up for lost time with visits and hospitalizations because my parents always expected me to do well at school.

I liked doing anything that stimulated me to grow, improve, and meet people. During the period when the illness was under control, I never had any significant problems doing things. Quite the opposite, even simple things were complicated when the drugs no longer covered me. I wanted to be a journalist.

People close to me said I was intelligent, willing, and determined. My family never really understood my illness; they often pretended nothing happened and demanded a lot. Very few close friends knew, and they always protected me a lot.

I sent and handed in a lot of CVs, but I was never discouraged, and I was lucky I found a good job immediately. I never mentioned my illness and was never asked anything about my health. My first experiences at work were good; I never took days off or sick leave and always did everything on my days out or when I wasn't working.

Treating epilepsy has always been difficult.

In the beginning, when I was 13, it seemed that the treatment was working, but I had to do a lot of check-ups because I wasn't always fully covered. When I was 18, they changed my medication, and I had Steven & Johnson's, which was terrible and very scary. Fortunately, I recovered, but it took me almost a year to recover physically. I took another drug with side effects and didn't take it regularly. I was fine without medication but had bad fits for five years. It was an ordeal'to find the proper treatment, then I finally found this drug, and it gave me an everyday, peaceful life. I also have side effects from it, but at least I have the seizures under control. I am confident I will also slowly resolve these things with the neurologist.

I felt terrible, wrong, uncomfortable, and different, and I had to prove that I was a good, "normal" person who performed better.

I am setting up my communication, event organization and image consultancy business. I am happy and satisfied. I have become self-employed. I am more aware of my potential and no longer held back by my insecurities related to the disease that I no longer hide.

The experience of the pandemic initially frightened me a lot because I have little immunity now due to my previous health problems and the availability of drugs. However, I could meet and collaborate with many people throughout Italy through digital tools.

I like my job, and I hope I can continue to do it without too many setbacks. I have learnt to reinvent myself. Sometimes, I am afraid of losing the balance I have found and not being able to do things again, but I try not to think about it. My relationship at work is good; I am very friendly by nature and by trade. They are beneficial, and I try to maintain good relations with everyone. The place of work is at a distance at present. People close to me say I am strong, determined, and strong-willed.

The epilepsy treatment is quite good; it allows me a good quality of life. I feel pretty well, hopefully always better. In balance with myself and my past.

Looking back on my career path, despite everything I am proud of, I would take better care of my health. I would like to have a more stable working life. To be well and have a family without fear of being sick and involving others.

Writing my story was liberating; it's a good initiative, thank you.

And thanks to you both, what reflective writers who have allowed us to enter your world made of dreams, becoming a teacher of human rights and image consultant. Gratitude to your resiliency despite having seen your CV rejected and having violated your human rights, not talking about your disability.

These two cases showed the massive difference between selling universal rights and utopian laws established by the United Nations and reality, a place full of dystopias. These two 40-year-old people made it and coped with it thanks to their relationships, families, good doctors, and their strengths. But it was, and it is incredibly enduring.

9.4 Children, The Future Generations

Because they are and will be our future, I would like to spend some time on the well-being and health of children, using the same methodology, the analysis of their rights. On November 20th, 1989, the Convention on the Rights of the Child and Adolescent was held, producing a treaty that includes all the rights of children, where the age is extended to 18 years.

9.4.1 *The Rights of Children and Adolescents*

From then on, a new view was given on children and adolescents as subjects with the rights to respect and fulfilment. Here are the ten main articles:

Right to play
All children have the right to play and enjoy themselves.
Right to food
All children have the right to food and to be adequately nourished.
Right to a home
All children have the right to have a home. A protected place where the child can live with understanding, love, and care.
Right to health
The right to health in children is one of the fundamental rights to which every child should have access.
The right to health is a compendium of physical, mental and social well-being, and even more so in children, who are more vulnerable to illness.
Right to education
All children have the right to education, regardless of gender, religion, nationality or other status. The state must do everything possible to ensure children have access to education.

9.4 Children, The Future Generations

The right to life and to have a family
The right of children to live and to have a family. Children, for the full development of their personality, need love and understanding. To grow up under the responsibility of their parents and in an atmosphere of affection.

Right to have a nationality
From birth, the child has the right to have a name and a surname.

Children's right to equality
Children's right to equality, regardless of race, religion or nationality. This aims to ensure that all children are treated equally, irrespective of their origin, the country they are from or the colour of their skin.

Children's right to express their opinion
The Convention on the Rights of the Child recognizes the freedom of children to express opinions freely, just like adults.

Children's right not to work
The child must be protected from neglect, cruelty, and exploitation. The child should not be allowed to work before an appropriate minimum age. Work is not allowed under the age of 13, and in Europe, work between the ages of 14 and 15 is provided as a small 'internship' in alternating school and work.

If we look back and think about child labor, European law has undoubtedly improved, and children have regained their childhood so well expressed in their first right to play. This is also thanks to the great movements of the early 1900s with Maria Montessori, Anna Freud, Sabine Spielrein, and Melanie Klein; however, only in 1989 were children acknowledged as subjects capable of expressing their own opinions. On paper. Forbidden now the phrases that many of our generation and previous generations grew up with: "Hush you who are a child" or "You don't know anything about this." Being kept in silence is a form of violence, and the more children are demanded to be quiet, the more likely they will use this behavior in educating their children. I don't question the boundaries and limits which must be taught to children as respect, inclusion, and loving emotions.

How capable are we adults of freely expressing our opinions? Self-expression is one of the first pillars for the mental well-being of the individual, and if it cannot be acted directly, it will be achieved through spoken word and an engaged audience. This art arises from unexpressed inner tension—that suffering that Jerome Bruner puts at the basis of narrative experience, an essential way of sublimating the conscious and unconscious messages we wish to communicate.

About "the right to have a family" the declaration of the rights of children and adolescents does not specify whom this family should be composed; however, two words that describe what qualities this family must set in motion: love and understanding, so that the child grows up in a dimension of affect and love, not of fear, silence, guilt. I wish also to highlight that *family* is a word which does not belong to the Natural Semantic Metalanguage, so it is not a universal. This means that in some cultural societies, as some nomadic tribes, the children (in NSM, the small ones), are loved, nourished and mentored by the adults and the senior (in NSM the big ones). Family, according to this linguistic approach could be considered as a conceptual superstructure. Love and "making the small ones feeling good" (in NSM language) is what matters.

9.4.2 Illness of Children and Play

Narratives of ill young children are rare, they are "better listened to" through their drawings. There is much evidence about the messages children can subliminally convey through the colors they use, whether bright or dark, how they fill in the empty paper, and how much pressure they give to their pencils. Perhaps this is why we create fairytales for them, based on the hero's journey or the natural cycle to explain life and death. I wonder whether they are deeply listened to in palliative care; maybe yes, because wonderful people work with children in this field.

Millions of children will die or whose lives are threatened by cancer, heart disease and genetic conditions. These children live with conditions that will shorten their lives and lead to death in childhood or early adulthood. All children with life-threatening and life-limiting conditions have the right to receive palliative care, which aims to ease the unpleasant symptoms of the illness or disease and improve the quality of life of the sick child and that child's family [16].

Rain, rain, go away.
Come again another day.
Little children want to play.
Rain, rain, go away.

Children's hospices are full of intense emotions, facing the utmost form of violence we could think of: chronic disease or the dying of a child. However, from what we know, they still play almost until the end or leave their toys to the child in the other room. No further words for this. Just the awareness that life is violent and unfair and that there is no sickness for children since they are all innocent. Stigma tends to become more apparent during adolescence. Let's learn from children who play until the end.

> The overwhelming nature of the illness cannot be approached 'y reality alone. Paradoxically, the illusion afforded by play is what allows reality to be integrated. Through play, the child can advance and retreat, draw near and pull away from the intense core. These tentative forays allow the child to contain and master the experience.

The fantastical world of the child at play should not be seen as avoidance of the truth because "*illusion is translucent, if not transparent, and thus reality shines through for both the child and the therapist even when not addressed directly by either*" [17].

Let the children play and move on in our world of adults. How much in our free time—which is a right sanctioned by the United Nations—do we use for play? Do we still know how to play? There are some extreme polarities on this topic. While I'm writing about the need to play, in Western schools, with over competition, hardly any time is dedicated to play. My heart is full of sorrow thinking about the denial of the right to education and going to university for women in Afghanistan and Iran.

Few know that playing is good for you! The purpose of this chapter is not to create a sort of "wonder effect" in relation to technical discoveries and the eloquently written codes of human rights and medical discoveries. It is to bring sustainable and light-hearted solutions to create well-being.

9.5 The Courses and Resources

These declarations continue as epic and necessary as the seventeen Sustainable Development Goals at another historic meeting in 2015 with the United Nations, which included the rights of the planet for the first time with equal opportunities as human beings (Fig. 9.2).

Likely, a spiral is one of the best symbols to represent health between violent and nonviolent times in history, starting from ancient civilizations and ending in our postmodern society. Reading the common traits between scientific discoveries, moral issues, wars, and illness, we began to question the motto *"Historia magistra vita"* to create well-being and health. Historians documented wars and battles of defense and offence, plagues for not closing their country harbors just in time, and famines because of crop devastations by insects. We, as a team, remarked overconfidence in the capacity of technological progress, as a repetition compulsion run by a Sapiens who perhaps is not very *Sapien*s, more a Not Sapiens animal.

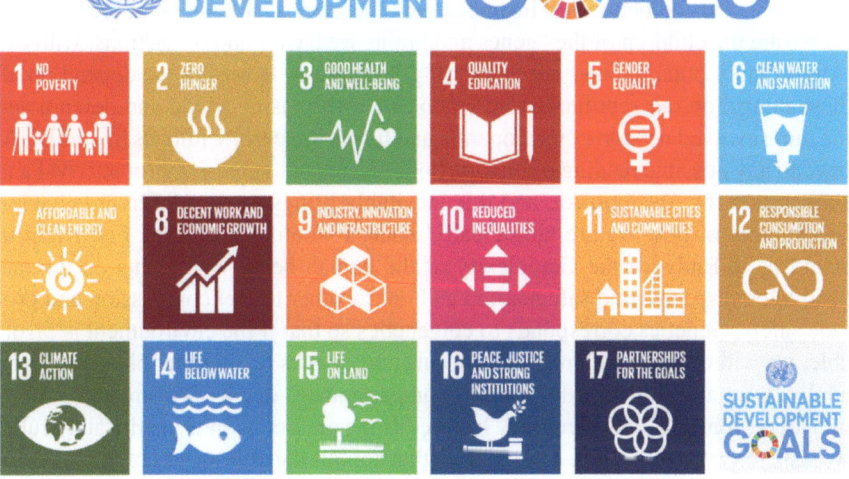

Fig. 9.2 Sustainable development goals of United Nations

9.6 Courses and Recurrences

The philosopher Giambattista Vico, from Naples, who lived between the 17th and 18th centuries, spoke courses and recurrences in history [18]. For Vico, studying history is a "new science," which must deal with identifying and documenting events and facts through the union of philosophy and philology. Above all, it must interpret them by searching for those ideal and eternal reasons, destined to constantly present themselves repetitively, albeit in different degrees, within all moments of history: the historical courses and recourses.

From Vico's perspective, human beings are always identical and not evolving, even in changing historical situations and behavior. What occurs again in history is only comparable by analogy to what has already happened. Vico defines recurrences not as a succession and repetition of the political forms of policies, but a succession and replay of all forms of human and social culture. Vico systematizes history as an event characterized by its intrinsic rationality. For the philosopher, it is a matter of grasping the norms and laws of that glorious and non-linear path that is the historical journey of nations.

It is as if, to find the meaning of events, Vico invites us to look beyond these facts, to grasp within history another invisible history—that of deeper reasons and ends. For Vico, the consequences of actions always go beyond the specific intentionality of men; humankind does more than he knows and is often not self-aware. Hence why history always seems to repeat itself.

We human beings have learned history enough and have the notions to be able to say stop to this immense and recursive brutality. Yet, it has not happened, even with historical culture. Why? According to Vico, there is a divine reason, but according to the latest discoveries of neuroscientists, there are biological reasons. And this is why we must face, despite all our human rights education, our "dark side." This continuous tension between selfishness and otherness is and will be perpetual.

We are the children of the "genes and brains we have," and our actions, with our extraordinary potential and our distressing limitations. However, we depend on all these things, on our reptilian brain, embodied within us to offend and defend, and the more evolved neocortex to cooperate and listen. We carry within us, in our DNA, beyond any possible reading of history, both vectors of aggressivity for survival and cooperation for development, and this inevitably brings us to a different behavior. Taking note of how we are biologically made, I would say that the first Right to Health is to Embrace the Complexity of the human being who wants on the one hand to be respected and safeguarded and on the other to feel compassion and provide safety. Genetics corresponds to epigenetics so that if the environment is favorable, we will develop children, adolescents and, thanks to neuronal plasticity, even adults, who are human, affectionate, compassionate, expressive, creative, determined, responsible, and eventually happier. If the environment is hostile and brutal, we will, unfortunately, have a population that applies the oldest parts of the brain for survival, offence, and defense, creating people who are sick and can cause tears and rifts between people by wars and terror.

How many forces of goodwill have traversed the millennia, and what wonder those spiritually dense 'sacred texts' of the grand declarations of human rights of recent years arouse in us? Two vectors, one for possession, one for distribution: too simplistic to divide into two; in between, there is a land of conciliation to give health, a balance between giving and having.

To come out of Utopia and Dystopia and simply be in the Place of the Real, improving the inequalities and lowering expectations. With lightness. With creative playfulness. Like the spiral of our galaxy, which presents circles in which the recurrences grow wider and wider to the initial position, to differentiate, because of the historical events, the Sapiens Neanderthal's understanding may be similar over the millennia but not the same.

9.7 Practice Time

9.7.1 Green Pass Between Utopic and Dystopic

In Francis Bacon's *New Atlantis*, Tommaso Campanella's *City of the Sun* and Thomas More's *Island of Utopia*, there are rules for creating well-being in society: education (including women, and we are in the 15th-16th-17th centuries), fair distribution of possessions, production for consumption and not for enrichment, and knowledge of various languages, even the ancient ones. In the *New Atlantis*, Bacon dwells on the need for scientific experimentation on dead bodies plants and the preservation of organs to create knowledge and well-being.

The "City of the Sun" (perhaps Sri Lanka) and the "New Atlantis," discovered by serendipity after a shipwreck in the South Seas, are utopian cities geographically located far away on separate islands, and difficult to reach. More's "Island of U-topia" (from *ou-topos*, no place, or perhaps a-topos, a good spot) is also located elsewhere that is difficult to define. Insularity means isolation from the earthly and corrupt world, distance and remoteness if not inaccessibility. All the people are happy in these islands or cities, and the governor's goal is the population's happiness. That is possible because no one has more than others. Envy, one of the capital vices which arises precisely from not having the luxuries of others, cannot germinate.

Campanella writes, "I was born to eradicate three extreme evils: / tyranny, sophistry, hypocrisy; [...] / Famines, wars, plagues, envy, deceit, / injustice, lust, sloth, disdain, / all of which are subject to those three great evils, / which have their root and foment in blind self-love, worthy son / of ignorance." Plague and famine are dependent on human behavior and are greatly intertwined with the establishment of absolutist governments, sophistry (i.e., rhetoric for its own sake aimed at a personal advantage, and hypocrisy (which can be understood today as denialism)—denying meaning to the things that happen, to nature with its phenomena and excesses.

The philosophers and scientists More, Bacon and Campanella, with their "heretical" and "illegal" political thoughts, spent part of their lives in prison. Thomas More was even beheaded for not having signed in favor of King Henry VIII. It is plausible that they dreamt of better, fairer worlds, where culture was seen as a common good and not as some form of power to manage the crowds, who had to remain ignorant and, in extreme cases, in misery.

Utopia is opposed to Dystopia (*dys*, bad and *topos*, place), the representation of an imaginary reality of the future, predictable based on highly negative present trends, in which an undesirable or frightening life is foreshadowed. Oppressive social or political phenomena characterize the society in conjunction with or as a consequence of dangerous environmental or technological conditions, including post-atomic world wars, meteorites, glaciation, and pandemics. The term "dystopian" originated, ironically, from a speech by the liberal economist Stuart Mill to recall the lack of freedom of movement, trade, and enrichment—an origin, then, far from the one of Utopia. The dystopian genre was successful in the last century because its imagery originated from a twofold trauma: on the one hand, the shock produced by the acceleration of technical and scientific progress, which lead to dehumanization and alienation, or the destruction of the environment and humanity itself; on the other hand, the trauma caused in the first half of the twentieth century by the rising of totalitarian regimes such as the Fascist, Nazi and Stalinist regimes, which largely inspired dystopian literature.

Among the great exponents is Aldous Huxley, author of *Brave New World* (1932), which describes a world based on eugenics and castes: they are tasked with performing get progressively harder, the lower their cast is. The alpha caste consists of individuals destined for leadership, meanwhile, the betas hold administrative positions requiring higher instruction but without command responsibilities. The gammas are created and trained to take on the most menial jobs and in very hard conditions without complaint. Delta children are conditioned through electric shocks to fear flowers and books to take on the most menial tasks; Epsilons, conditioned from childhood to hate nature and the countryside and love cities and factories, take on the ugliest jobs and under the harshest conditions. In general, all individuals are mentally conditioned to conform to the role they will play in society.

Another exponent of the dystopic genre is George Orwell. Quotations from his book 1984 were favorites of people opposed to the COVID-19 pandemic lockdown and the continuous laws that restricted people's movement. In George Orwell's book 1984, we follow the main protagonist, Winston Smith, as he navigates London in what he believes to be 1984. Working for the Ministry of Truth, he spends his days as a journalist altering news articles and erasing the past. This is the world he lives in. A world in which the past, present, and future are managed by "Big Brother" and members of the "Ingsoc Inner Party," the governing ideology of the Oceania region. In Oceania, privacy does not exist. Secret telescreens and microphones are everywhere—in the streets, workplaces, restaurants and especially in homes. They watch you and listen to you. All that is private is your thoughts; even those are illegal if they don't obey Ingsoc's beliefs. It's called "thoughtcrime." Thoughtcrime describes a person's politically unorthodox thoughts, such as beliefs and doubts contradicting Ingsoc's principles.

In an online post, the author—clearly against lockdowns and forced restriction of personal freedom—states,

> 2020 has seen a wave of pulling wrong thoughts from the minds of others. Articles and social media posts that don't align with the story we are fed are quickly censored and taken down under the context that spreading false information is a major safety concern for our society's health and well-being during a crisis. [...] [People] are losing their jobs and careers, and their reputations are being tarnished because of cancel culture and essentially *1984's* thoughtcrime.

There are many other posts like this on the net, just type 'Orwell and pandemic' into Google, and you will find a whole host of these kinds of comments. While it is true that many have lost their jobs during the lockdowns, it is also true that the Green Pass and Covid-Free islands created another dystopian narrative.

I am reminded of two dystopian science fiction movies released before the "dystopian film" of the pandemic that we have been living on and within our skin since February 21st, 2020. These films are not about viral contagions or stories that set themselves up as prophetic of viruses that have escaped from the Wuhan labs. "Elysium" and "Snowpiercer" are titles that spring up in my mind as two possible representations of the current global situation, not only in our little ol'Europe, which is not very capable of signing proper contracts with some pharmaceutical companies to get vaccines, but also in other countries and continents, where are already counting the deaths due to lack of access to treatment, respirators, oxygen, and finally the vaccine.

"Elysium" is a 2013 film starring Jodie Foster and Matt Dammon, directed by the South African Canadian Neil Blomkamp. In 2154, humankind is divided into two castes: a handful of aristocrats. Who live on an enormous space station called Elysium, orbiting around the earth, luxurious, futuristic and equipped with a perfect terrestrial ecosystem; and the poor, the vast majority, live on planet earth, now overpopulated, highly polluted and almost uninhabitable because of the state of significant decay. The government of Elysium establishes stricter and stricter laws against immigration to preserve the luxury and well-being of the privileged few who live there and to stop by shooting down with missiles the unauthorized ships the people who, from earth, continually try to reach the station illegally immigrants. A worker on Earth, Max (Matt Dammon), is exposed to a massive dose of gamma radiation, which, according to the medical robots serving the poor inhabitants of the planet, will kill him within five days. Max's only hope is to reach Elysium quickly, where he can use the highly advanced medical capsules, which can heal any illness or physical damage in seconds, even severe ones. However, he is confronted by Jodie Foster, chief of police of Elysium. I will not reveal how the sequel unfolds, but it is clear that the whole film is about the accessibility of technologically advanced treatments.

"Snowpiercer," is a 2013 film directed by Bong Joon-ho (also director of "Parasite"), based on the graphic novel *Le Transperceneige*, a post-apocalyptic science fiction comic. The year is 2031 and takes place in a world decimated by a new ice period caused by failed experiments to stop global warming. A group of 2100 people remain alive inside a train, the "Snowpiercer," which continues to move around the earth and obtains the necessary energy through a perpetual engine. The train is a microcosm of human society divided into social classes. The poorest live crammed into the last carriages, where they feed exclusively on protein bars made from insects, the richest live in the front carriages. Informed of how the upper classes live by people in prison at the back of the train, the "nobodies" start a revolution. The theme of food, care, and available space is the film's leitmotif. Interestingly, the original thinking (the earth is slowly recovering and becoming habitable again) is in the wagon of the desperate. At the same time, the wealthy classes—in truth, many of them are the economic investors in the train—and their children continue to believe, "Big Brother style," in the sophistry that the train is the best of all possible worlds.

Returning to the 2020–2021 pandemic, the report by Michael Marmot, Professor of Epidemiology at the University College of London and Director of the Institution of Health Equity, came out in December 2020. Though the report, titled "Build Back Fairer," focuses primarily on the UK it may prove to be paradigmatic for other countries. Again, in an April 2021 interview in The Guardian, Marmot confirms that the pandemic and the associated social response have amplified social and economic inequalities from early childhood, education, employment, having enough money to live on, housing, and community. It also showed even steeper social gradients in mortality rates and surprisingly high mortality rates among people from ethnic minority groups. Much of this excess can be attributed to poverty or lack of access to care [19].

The whole pandemic has been immense burden to bear not only for our bodies but also for our minds and souls in terms of access to care, from the availability of oxygen, masks, personal protective equipment, and available beds to the current case of vaccination, which is highly delayed in Italy (considered of the five countries in the world most affected by the pandemic). The Green Pass—which stated that only vaccinated people or people who have had COVID-19 could travel—put us in a dystopian place (prompted discrimination). Given the uncertainty, scientists objected to giving the green light for travel to people who tested negative two days before their trip.

The vaccination calendar, except for health professionals, has been full of mistakes. Only at the end of March, after vaccinating professors, some judges, and administrative staff in the public administration, they have begun to vaccinate the fragile population over 80 and younger people in vulnerable situations. Millions of people in Italy have been waiting for the first injection of vaccine to obtain a Green Pass, and in the meantime, the government, to boost tourism, is creating "Covid-free islands" like Capri and Panarea (places for wealthy people, in my opinion). Vaccines will be given more slowly to the "normal population," but faster to those who can afford recreating this kind of paradise, a vaccination resort.

The younger generation paid an undignified price because they were the last to receive the vaccine, so they were seriously exposed to the risk of not finding jobs or not being able to travel and/or learn for much longer. Another remark about the islands-- the COVID-free slogan has been created to boost tourism. The entire population will be vaccinated on islands such as the Aeolian Islands or Capri, regardless of the vulnerability risk. Holidays on the island will have a utopian flavor for those who bought them through monetary wealth, an idea that contradicts Bacon, Campanella, and Mores' description of a utopian island. On the other end of the spectrum, unvaccinated people still pay and will pay a price for freedom of movement and opportunities, young people especially, with fewer chances for employment because they are not yet vaccinated in a society that is even more dystopian for them. The Green Pass should have been implemented when most of the population was equally vaccinated, taking into consideration herd immunity as a potential safety factor.

Access to the Covid-19 vaccination in January 2022 in Africa was as follows: out of more than 9 billion vaccine doses produced, Africa has only received approximately 540 million (about 6% of all COVID vaccines, despite having 17% of the world's population) and administered 309 million doses. Less than 10% of Africans are fully vaccinated. The COVID narrative on vaccination is a case that is still paradigmatic to remember. However, these inequalities are still here today: there are ethical problems with access to health, which enforces the slow violence that emerged from desperation as life-sustaining conditions eroded.

Have you ever found yourself in a Utopian situation? What about a Dystopian condition? What kind of communication did you have with the inhabitants of the two places? Please forgive the extreme polarizations. Where did you feel you belonged? This is a significant existential clue.

9.7.2 *Right to Play to Lightness for Children, Adults, and Older People*

I would like to expand on the importance of play in adults by presenting a study from Switzerland, Germany, and the UK that found that playing at any age generates positive health outcomes.

9.7.3 *Playfulness*

Adult playfulness is a personality trait that allows people to frame or reframe everyday situations in such a way as to experience them as fun, intellectually stimulating or personally interesting. Various research supports the idea that playfulness is associated with pursuing an active lifestyle. While playful children are typically described as active, there is limited knowledge on whether playfulness in adults is also associated with physical activity. We used a multifaceted model that allows us to distinguish between other-oriented, carefree, intellectual and extravagant playfulness. To fill this gap in the literature, we conducted two studies on the associations of playfulness with health, activity and fitness. The main focus of the first study was to compare evaluations of self (N = 529) and other acquaintances (N = 141). We tested the association of self and peer-reported playfulness with physical activity, fitness and health behaviors reported by self and peers. Good convergence of playfulness was found between self and peer evaluations (between r = 0.46 and 0.55, all p < 0.001). The data show that self- and peer evaluations are differentially associated with physical activity, fitness and healthy behavior. For example, self-evaluation of playfulness shares 3% of the variance with self-evaluation of physical fitness and 14% with active lifestyle seeking. The second study provides data on the association between the self-assessment of playfulness and objective measures of physical fitness (hand and forearm strength, lower body muscle strength and endurance, cardio-respiratory capacity, back and leg flexibility, hand and finger dexterity) using a sample of N = 67 adults. Self-reported playfulness was associated with lower heart rate at baseline and activity (climbing stairs) and faster recovery heart rate (correlation coefficients were between −0.19 and −0.24 for overall playfulness). Overall, the second study confirmed the first study's results, showing positive associations between playfulness and objective indicators of physical fitness (mainly cardio-respiratory fitness). The results represent a starting point for future studies on the relationships between playfulness, health, activity and physical fitness (Proyer 2018).

But beyond the improved physical strength resulting from movement games, what gives well-being through play is the willingness to explore and accept complexity:

> Playfulness is a variable of individual differences that allows people to frame or reframe everyday situations in such a way as to experience them as fun, and/or intellectually stimulating, and/or personally interesting. Those at the high end of this dimension seek out and establish situations where they can interact playfully with others (e.g., playful teasing, shared play activities) and use their playfulness even in difficult situations to resolve tensions (e.g., in social interactions or work-related contexts). Playfulness is also associated with a preference for complexity over simplicity and a preference for—and a liking of—unusual activities, objects and topics or individuals' [20].

Here are a few examples of adults' playfulness: 'playing with new ideas', 'breaking out of established patterns,' 'expressing one's emotions to a partner with a game,' 'swimming against the tide—to the letter,' 'making friends with people outside the usual circle,' 'creating one's expressive style,' 'using playfulness to cheer up others,' 'a playful approach to learning new things', 'being able to smile about what happens.' In fact, the more I write down these examples, the more I realize that play makes the brain more neuro-plastic and creates new synaptic connections. They are games of creativity and cheerfulness with very little competition. That is why they give existential well-being.

Play momentarily removes us from emotional heaviness, and undoubtedly invites us to lightness, as Calvin taught us in his *Six Memos for the Next Millennium* [21]:

> *I want to close this lecture by recalling a short story by Kafka, Der Kübelreiter (The Bucket Rider). It is a short story in the first person, written in 1917, and its starting point is an authentic situation in that winter of war, the most terrible for the Austrian empire: the lack of coal. The narrator goes out with an empty bucket in search of coal for the stove. On the way, the bucket acts as his horse. Indeed, he lifts it to close-up height and carries it convincing as if on the back of a camel. The coalman's shop is underground, and the bucket rider is too high up; he finds it hard to understand himself by the man who would be ready to accommodate him, while his wife does not want to hear him. He begs them to give him a shovelful of the cheapest coal, even though he cannot pay immediately. The coalman's wife unties her apron and chases away the intruder as she would chase a fly. The bucket is so light that it flies away with its rider until it is lost beyond the Ice Mountains. Many of Kafka's short stories are mysterious, and this one is particularly so. Perhaps Kafka just wanted to tell us that searching for some coal on a cold wartime evening turns into a*

wandering knight's quête, a caravan's crossing in the wilderness, a magical flight, to the simple rocking of the empty bucket. But the idea of this empty bucket that lifts you above the level where the help and even the selfishness of others are to be found, the empty bucket a sign of deprivation and longing and searching that elevates you to the point where your humble prayer can no longer be answered, – opens the way to endless reflections. I had spoken of the shaman and the hero of fairy tales, of the suffered privation that transforms into lightness and allows you to fly into the realm where every lack will be magically compensated. I had spoken of the witches who flew on humble do-nothings like a bucket. But the hero of this Kafka tale does not appear to be endowed with shamanic or witch-like powers, nor does the realm beyond the Ice Mountains appear to be one in which the empty bucket will find something to fill. Especially since if it were complete, it would not allow flying. So, straddling our bucket, we will face the new millennium without hoping to find anything more in it than what we will be able to bring—Lightness, for example, whose virtues this bucket has sought to illustrate.

9.7.4 Alignment or Misalignment for a More Sustainable Ecosystem

When we speak about a healthcare ecosystem, we mean the complexity of human beings and their roles as healthcare providers, humans dedicated to giving health, well-being, and comfort. This can be achieved through narrative medicine: listening to the needs of the individuals within the realm of possibilities—listening also to the needs of the doctors as persons and not just as roles. The juxtaposition process invites us to keep in mind two or more things which might not converge at the same time: a sewing needle to patch together pluralities of opinion, opposed to scissors that serve to oversimplify reality.

We are very aware that this world is polluted by the over prescription of medications, a quick and fix system, selling, with a loud voice, the idea that there is a remedy for every discomfort. As Doctor Dulcamara in the opera "Elisir D'Amore" ("The Love Elixir"), written by Gaetano Donizetti, he sells his bottled "cure-all" to the townspeople, including love potions. His "elixir," which is just cheap red wine, is bought at a price of his choosing. And sometimes, by chance, it succeeds, especially with young people. But we know this kind of Elixir might have a temporary placebo effect that will fade. Quick fixes, as we know, do not apply to most types of situational discomforts.

Alignment in the listening to the needs of all actors on stage is warranted: sometimes it is achieved, sometimes not, but always has a long-term effect.

It was extraordinarily achieved in the first months of the COVID-19 age, those darkest days, going to February, March, and April 2020. ISTUD administered a survey to patients, caregivers, and doctors, asking for a definition for this unknown virus, to which it was unanimously agreed upon that the virus was "a monster." A monster is an aberration from nature, something hidden, invisible, lethal, and dangerous. The alignment was complete, apart from a few deniers, the same people who are now deniers of climate change, there was a global effort by everyone in this ecosystem. Most citizens respected the lockdown rules, some shielding themselves, doctors and nurses were risking their lives to "try" to save other lives without any elixir tool, and personal protective equipment was handcrafted when not available.

Moving away from COVID-19, let's enter another topic, which might also be driven by the social pressure of our contemporary life: depression. Ninety-six narratives from Italians with major depression (36), their caregivers (27), and psychiatrists (33) were collected in Italian (and therefore word clouds were built in Italian), and here the Italian words used at the prompt "I was feeling…" ("mi sentivo"). [22].

The word cloud from the patient with depression narrative at "I was feeling…" gave the following picture (Fig. 9.3):

The word cloud from the doctor's narratives, under the prompt "He/S was feeling," gave the following picture (Fig. 9.4):

Doctors look at the patients more from an emotional point of view, using the Italian words such as "triste" and "tristezza" (sad and sadness), and "*senza speranza*" meaning hopeless, also referred to the "inadequate" (inadequate) category, in the realm of the not being able to do.. It looks like doctors are not always aware of the "real condition" reported in the patients' words like *solo/sola (lonely)* and *perso/persa* (lost). It was shockingly revealed that the depression was barely perceived by caregivers, people who live close to them.

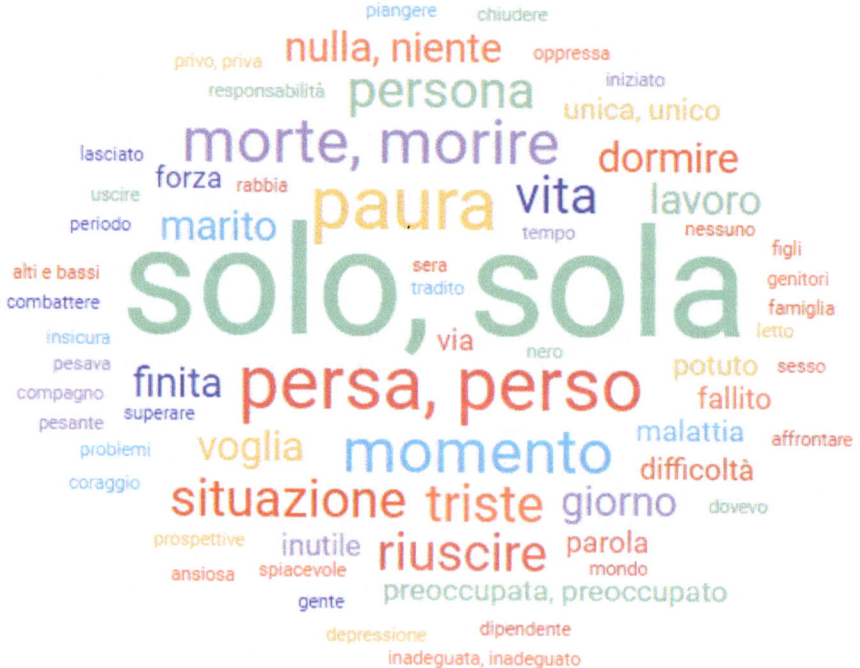

Fig. 9.3 Word cloud of patients' feelings

9.7 Practice Time

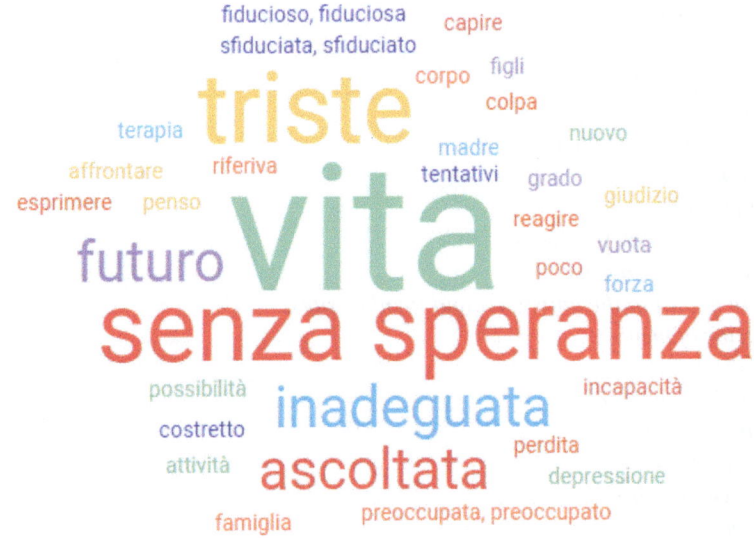

Fig. 9.4 Word cloud of doctors' perception of patients' feelings

Beyond this, the words "morire and morte" (to die and dead) are only written in the patients' narratives. The healthcare professionals, possibly unable to handle the possible risk of suicide, replaced the words to die or death with *"senza speranza,"* hopeless.

The collected narratives suggested that, while patients are in the "to be" dimension, as indicated by the words "solo" and "sola" encoded in our cultural script of depression, carers are in the "to do" dimension, more based on "performance adequacy," as in DSM-5 written by the American Psychiatric Association; this difference could explain the loss of reciprocal understanding, creating the feeling of loneliness. This is a notable misalignment of which all people curing people with depression should be informed: but not only for severe depression, also for every daily "nervous breakdown" [23].

In this ecosystem, while the patients whisper about loneliness or confusion, the carers reply with an assessment of "inadequacy" and "hopelessness." Don't we taste a mildly bitter flavor of judgment? Could this ecosystem be less of a threat while creating a better intimacy with the courage to ask questions such as "Lonely? What do you mean by being or feeling lonely?"; "Confused, in which sense?"; "How could I help you? What could help you?"; "Is there anything you might like?"; "How could I help you and the people around you to feel less lonely"? Perhaps just listening to the patient's words, making room for "awkward silence," silence has a sound too. We have no need for more quick and easy fixes like Dulcamara's Elixir, instead active listening and creative thinking will improve the alignment and healing among those living in the ecosystem.

And now, what are our feelings about relaxing, getting away from sad pitches, and reading Dulcamara's aria:

Hear, hear, or rust;
Be careful; do not breathe.
I already suppose and imagine
That as you know, me
What a great doctor I am,
Encyclopedic doctor
Called Dulcamara,
The virtue of which preclaces,
And the infinite portents
They are known to the universe...and to other sites.
Benefactor of men,
Fixing diseases,
In a few days, I clear,
I sweep the hospitals,
And health to sell
For the whole world, I want to.
Buy it, buy it,
I'll give it to you for a while.
This is the odontalgic
Wonderful liquor,
Of mice and bedbugs
Mighty destroyer.
Whose certificates
Authentic, branded
Touch, see and read
I'll do it to each one.
For this specific mine,
Sympathetic, prolific,
...
In a short week
More than a distressed widow
To cry ceased.
Or you rigid matrons,
Antiaging craved?
Your wrinkles are uncomfortable
With it, you delete.
You want damsels,
Well, smooth to have the skin?
You, young gallant,
Forever having lovers?
Buy my specific,
I'll give it to you for a while.
The paralytics move;
He sends the apoplectic,
Asthmatic, asthmatic,

The hysterics, the diabetics,
Heals tympanites...
You will tell me: how much does it cost?
How much is the bottle worth?
One hundred coins? ... thirty? ... twenty? ...
No...nobody is dismayed.
To prove my happiness
Yes, welcome friend,
I want you, or good people,
A regal shield.

References

1. https://www.un.org/en/un-chronicle/world-population-surpasses-8-billion-what-are-implications-planetary-health-and
2. Iain MGC. The master and his emissary: The Divided Brain and the Making of the Western World. Yale University Press; 2019.
3. https://unctad.org/system/files/official-document/wir2022_en.pdf
4. Sigmund F. Civilization and its discontents. London: The Hogarth Press and the Institute of Psycho-Analysis; 1972.
5. Hannah A. Eichmann in Jerusalem: a report on the banality of evil. Viking Press; 1963.
6. Herbert M. One-dimensional man: studies in the ideology of advanced industrial society. Beacon Press; 1991.
7. Calvino I. Le Città Invisibili. Giulio Einaudi Edition; 1972.
8. Nixon R. Slow violence and the environmentalism of the poor. Cambridge, MA: Harvard University Press; 2011.
9. WHO. World Health Statistics 2023. Monitoring Health for SDGs; 2023. www.who.org
10. Marcelo S, et al. Are we ready for a true biopsychosocial–spiritual model? The many meanings of "spiritual". Medicines (Basel). 2017;4(4):79.
11. https://www.fao.org/3/cb4476en/cb4476en.pdf
12. Chan A. https://www.huffpost.com/entry/america-never-abolished-slavery_b_6777420
13. Yuval H. Sapiens—a brief history of humankind. Penguin Random House UK; 2011.
14. https://www.who.int/standards/classifications/international-classification-of-functioning-disability-and-health
15. Merleau-Ponty M. Phenomenology of perception. Taylor & Francis Ltd.; 2013.
16. Boucher S, et al. The role of play in children's palliative care. Children. 2014;1(3):302–17.
17. Association for Children's Palliative Care (ACT) Royal College of Paediatrics and Child Health (RCPCH). A guide to the development of children's palliative care services: report of the joint working party. Bristol: ACT/RCPCH; 1997.
18. Vico GB. La Scienza nuova. 1743.
19. https://www.health.org.uk/publications/build-back-fairer-the-covid-19-marmot-review
20. Proyer F. 2017. https://www.researchgate.net/publication/311631718_A_new_structural_model_for_the_study_of_adult_playfulness_Assessment_and_exploration_of_an_understudied_individual_differences_variable.
21. Italo C. Six memos for the next millennium. Penguin Books Ltd; 2016.
22. Chesi P, Mencacci C, et al. Multicentre narrative research on major depression to integrate the experiences of patients, their caregivers and healthcare providers in Italy. BMJ. 2022;12(10):e052744.
23. https://www.psychiatry.org/psychiatrists/practice/dsm

Chapter 10
Multiple Intelligences to A Healthcare Wonderland

People who boast about their IQ are losers.—Stephen Hawkings

The pandemic, the European war, the shortage of resources, and the wealth inequalities subjected us to an immense test of reinventing ourselves and our society.

There are so many know-it-all's, so many reactive, offensive and defensive impulse opinions in healthcare, in the media, among the citizens, a "mountain" of violent news to process, and so little brilliant thinking that gives us and the future generation the possibility of hope for a new beginning. We need beyond technical STEM discipline also more innovative and more ethical intelligence.

In this last chapter, inspired by a work undertaken with students in a Master at ISTUD for preparing an e-book called "Tips to be brilliant" [1]. The book analyses concepts and go through a journey in multiple intelligences developed by Howard Gardner describing the qualities of men and women who are considered universally as geniuses [2]. A few of the names discussed are Dante, Leonardo Da Vinci, Jane Austen, Luis Pasteur, Ignaz Semmelweiss, Emily Dickinson, Nikola Tesla, Vincent Van Gogh, Coco Chanel and the Beatles. Now let us investigate together what we may learn from them and to improve our well-being.

10.1 How Do We Define Intelligence?

Capacity for logic, understanding, abstract thinking, reasoning, intuition, and adaptation? It is generally measured by the Intelligence Quotient, which gives a standard value of 100 with a deviation from normality generally of plus or minus 15. The Flynn effect, named after James Flynn, who discovered this trend across countries over the last century, describes the increase in the value of the average IQ of the population over the years. For this reason, it was considered by him to be independent of culture. To be more specific, Flynn observed a steady increase of about 3 points in the international IQ score every decade. Unfortunately, however, his euphoria was dampened in 2004, when, based on some empirical research, the University of Oslo noticed that the Flynn effect had diminished between 1970 and 1993. In the following years, it was confirmed that the trend had reversed, and from one year to the next, the international IQ decreased by an average of 0.25–0.50 points.

Trying to take an IQ test (I took two tests), one finds that the questions are related only to logical deductive, mathematical, and visual-spatial intelligence. One, therefore, wonders whether this instrument is valid and suitable for capturing genius, art, imagination, cooperation, intuition, ethics, and love for oneself and one's health, for others and for nature. That is why Howard Gardner has come to our aid, trying to widen the limit of the single tool of the Intelligence Quotient.

Gardner proposes this list of intelligences:

- Linguistic intelligence ("intelligence of speech")
- Logical-mathematical intelligence ("brilliant in numerical reasoning")
- Spatial intelligence ("intelligence of images")
- Bodily-kinesthetics intelligence ("brilliant in the use of the body")
- Musical intelligence ("brilliant in listening to and creating music")
- Interpersonal intelligence ("brilliant with people")
- Intrapersonal intelligence ("brilliant with oneself")
- Naturalistic intelligence ("brilliant with nature")

Gardner also includes an existential intelligence encompassing a spiritual and ethical sphere.

However, there are many more intelligences, as we will find out: among them, the capability of resilience, loving, decision-making, patience, and perseverance.

Please, reader, follow me to investigate another genius girl: Beth Harmon, a character created by Walter Tevis, an American novelist of the last century. Then, we will "use" Beth with the other real-life famous geniuses, from Dante to the Beatles, and eventually to our living times for promoting wellness and de-escalating conflicts.

10.1.1 **The Queen's Gambit**: *Beth Harmon*

Beth Harmon is the protagonist of Walter Tevis' book *The Queen's Gambit*, better known to the Italian public as *The Queen of Chess*. The work, written in 1983 by Walter Tevis, "a tribute to brainly women" as the author declares to The New York Time, has been "translated" into a beloved series by the Netflix sequel of the same title, where the chess queen, Beth Harmon, is played by three different Beths: the first, a little girl, who after losing her mother to suicide is placed in an orphanage, and meets a janitor, Mr. Scheibel, who secretly teaches her to play chess. The second representing her adolescence spent with her adoptive family that ends up separating. Finally, Beth- now a young woman- embodied by actress Anya Taylor-Joy, who has enchanted the world with her brown eyes and impeccable looks, must play a mental battle against herself. Beth is pretty- not beautiful, yet this means nothing

10.1 How Do We Define Intelligence?

to her as she later is recognized by a global audience as a genius, winning the world championship in chess.

Indeed, the writer knew how to play chess well, but beyond knowing how to play chess, imagined and recreated with language the behaviour and qualities of a genius from childhood, as in the case of the very successful Beth Harmon:

> *Gym was bad, and volleyball was worst...Beth could never hit the ball right. Most girls laughed and shouted when they played, but Beth never did...Beth tried it a few more times and did it better...After a few times, it got to be easy...Beth worked on it over the next week, and after that, she did not mind volleyball at all.*

It wasn't that Beth didn't mind playing volleyball at all, she endured it until she no longer suffered playing volleyball. But Beth didn't like it. There was no necessary drive, that pleasure principle on which one can choose things to love. She applied herself but took no joy from it, having found herself in an environment as cold, uncaring and gloomy as an orphanage in the 1950s, in the conservative USA led by President Eisenhower.

Here is Beth's first real interaction with Mr. Sheibel:

> *"You should be upstairs with the others." "I don't want to be with the others" She said. "I want to know what game you're playing." "It's called chess"..." Will you teach me"?" Girls don't play chess"...Mr. Sheibel was silent for a while. Then he pointed at the one with what looked like a smashed lemon on top. "This one"? ... Her heart leapt—answering, "On the diagonals."*

Beth observes the janitor playing alone and begins to "guess" some of its rules, including the fact that the bishop ("the one with the crushed lemon on top") moves diagonally. Mr. Scheibel, reminds her that she should be with the other girls at the orphanage. Beth refuses because she knows, with certainty, that she is attracted to this game, despite it being unsuitable for girls during a time period in the US in which a woman's value was based in her beauty and role as a mother.

Let's move on now to real-life examples. Emily Dickinson said "NO" to the school that wanted her to be a Christian and to marriage, Jane Austin to marriage, Nikola Tesla to the priesthood that his father wanted to impose on him, Ignaz Semmelweiss to the study of Law chosen by his father who left because he fell in love with Medicine. Because all of them preferred something else.

That evening, *"The noises had already faded into the white, harmonious background. Beth lay happily in bed, playing chess."*

Beth has understood what gives her happiness: it is not playing volleyball, it is not being with others, but it is *imagining a chess game* in her head.

Mr. Scheibel, having explained other rules of the game to her, appraises her talent once he is beaten. He then calls another chess master, and Beth wins them both. The master, Mr. Ganz, gives her a doll that Harmon throws in the wastebasket. She wanted a chess set, not a doll for little girls, and she will only have it for years once she wins her first prize once adopted by a couple whose husband disappears, leaving the alcohol-addicted wife alone to care for Beth. Without a real chessboard, Beth plays using memory to visualize a chess board, a bit like Dante imagined his Comedy, Tesla imagined alternating electric power and the machinery to produce it, and Coco Chanel did not paint sketches of her clothes on paper but created them on a mannequin. On the other hand, even Einstein had seen, not written down, the theory of relativity. Then, he had to write it down to convince the scientific community that he wanted nothing to do with equating and uniting matter and energy (a concept that Tesla had already anticipated).

Mrs. Wheatley, the adoptive mother, having realized her talent, also stands by her to get out of misery together agreeing to receive 10% of the winnings. When Mrs. Wheatly dies, Beth sinks into a void of alcohol and tranquillizers. Although she is a US champion, one Sunday morning, her brain is half-destroyed by addiction; she loses a match in her old homeland, Kentucky, to a young boy against whom it should have been impossible and ridiculous to lose against.

There are four elements that pull her out of the nightmare of disappearing. Realizing that her visual-spatial intelligence, her imagination, is no longer enough. This awareness, a demonstration of *intrapersonal introspective intelligence*, is acquired during her visit as an adult to the orphanage for Mr. Scheibel's funeral. It is in this moment that she comes to understand the headmistress's roughness and the janitor's tenderness, who kept newspaper cuttings with Beth's photos in the basement as she lifted pictures of her many trophies won around the world. It was seeing the narrowness of this cramped, almost closet-like, cupboard that led her to the awareness that if she had been born into another family, they might have acknowledged her earlier as a unique talent, sent her straight away to study chess, not punished her by taking away the thing she loved most and at which she was brilliant. Through this introspection, she understands, with enormous suffering, that she did everything almost on her own. She also understood why she self-harmed so much using alcohol and tranquillizers. Maybe it is through knowing ourselves, our biography, as Socrates taught in his *gnōthi sauton*, "know thyself," that we can de-escalate self-violence.

The second element is the *need for continuous education*. Given Beth's circumstances she often had to rely heavily on herself, taking the initiative to teach herself. For example, she studies the ramblings of the chess magazines she steals, and she begins to study to inform herself to fill the in the gaps in her knowledge and skillset. Beth knows there were years when she should have studied something else, but other occupations stole that time from her.

Beth puts forth much effort towards the competitions while her competitors are out sightseeing because she feels she must apply herself much more than someone who is "born learned." She studies her moves and the games of those who will be her competitors. And she studies Russian to understand what the world chess champions say and how they think. Dante was also a self-taught artist who spoke Latin but lacked Greek as a classical study and perhaps devoted himself, in spite of his depression (his "dark forest"), to the launch of a new language, the "Italian vulgar." He grasps the Italian he hears on the streets, writes it down, and gives it to us in his Commedia. Thanks to the continuous application and effort, Beth succeeds in *riveder le Stelle* ("seeing the stars again"). *Perseverance* is another form of intelligence not mentioned by Gardner. She understands that talent alone is never enough.

The third element is *asking for help with her interpersonal intelligence*. Beth uses discernment to ask the right people for help at the correct times. One morning, as she is regretfully self-medicating, she decides to seek out an early childhood friend from the orphanage, Jolene, who remains a wonderful friend. Jolene, studying and working as a physical education teacher, gets Beth into shape and stays close to her. When Beth admits to not knowing how to win the Russian championship, she trains with all the best champions available. As explained to her, this is very rare in America, where people work more in isolation.

In contrast, it was a typical habit for the Russians, where everyone rehearsed together for days before competitions. Individual play in the USA and team play in Russia and this is the reason why there are so many chess champions in the latter country. Again, Leonardo asked for help through his letter to be received at court by Ludovico il Moro, not only as a painter, but as an engineer of war machines for defence. Pasteur asked for money from Napoleon III for his laboratory to become the *Institut Pasteur*. And the Beatles, who, with their group equation $1 + 1 + 1 = \infty$, invented an impressive number of musical and textual motifs.

And then there is the Fourth Element of Power to Succeed, perhaps the most significant one: when Beth "is at an impasse" during the games, she does not know what to move; she is on the defensive; she is in danger of losing; in this instant she *"no longer feels the need to win the other," no longer feels the competition of war.* Instead of looking the "opponent in the face," she focuses on the aesthetics of the chessboard, the moves, and the sense of pleasure and playfulness she derives from the game. The other no longer exists. She plays honour chess, because she loves it. Thus, she wins.

The fourth element is intelligence of loving, fascination, and Voluntas ("willingness"), and enjoyment. This quality is present in all the intelligent people mentioned before, that is, not only the ability to say "NO," but also, to pursue tirelessly to cultivate one's passion.

> *Sunlight filtered through the trees on her...When she stopped at his table, he looked at her inquisitively, but his face had no recognition. She sat behind the black pieces and said carefully in Russian, "Would you like to play chess?*

These are the last lines of Walter Tevis's novel. The pleasure of chess, even with a perfect stranger who does not know she is the brilliant world champion.

10.1.2 The Voluntas

I used Beth Harmon as a symbol of genius with the limitations of a literary character. However, she effectively shifts the focus from lived biographies to a fantastic character many know and admire. I could have chosen Odysseus, the multifaceted man, and Sherlock Holmes, the connoisseur of the tiniest clues. However, she captivated and chose me, not only for the Netflix TV series *The Queen's Gambit* but for Tevis's novel's dry, emotional prose. I do not begrudge the intellectuals, the lost geniuses, the living geniuses, and the geniuses of future generations.

From the analysis of the previously mentioned individuals, including fictional ones like Beth Harmon, Voluntas appears to come first in the qualities of a genius. What is Voluntas?- the etymology derives from the Latin 'Velle' meaning to want. In this, voluntas implies the meaning of desiring, of choosing, of something that originates spontaneously, and of pleasure. Perhaps of all the possible synonyms, the term that attracts the most attention is the adverb "spontaneously," the roots of which tell us that it is precisely something that comes forth in space without nudging, coercion, or manipulation. It's an act of freedom. It is a call to act spontaneously, without too many calculations of return, of advantage, without excesses of rationalization.

The word "Want" is one of 64 terms included in the Semantic Natural Metalanguage (MSN), the metalanguage that exists universally in the planet's languages. Other words include "I," "You," "Body," "Thinking," "feeling" (as in emotions, "to feel"), "Knowing," "Power" ("to be able to"), "Doing," "Happening," "Living" and "Dying" ...Existential issues. There is no human being who does not want, aspire, or desire if the map of words is an expression of how we are and what we think. We read that the significant absence among these universal words is "Duty": we can construct it by assembling these words into the phrase 'I want you to do this thing'.

10.1.3 Self-realization: The Reason for Living

Again, concerning the word Voluntas, I would like it to be distinct from that more adequately described by Arthur Schopenhauer, who opposed the need to express Voluntas. Schopenhauer stated that humanity's unhappiness lies in chasing after its desires. He had embraced Eastern philosophies aimed at zeroing one's desires. As Voluntas, speaking of a subject as powerful as a genius, we do not mean to desire a new house, a new social status, or more incredible wealth. This willingness, in our sense, is to realize what we genetically (what we are bearers of) and epigenetically (the effect the context has on us) came into the world for. It would be like taking away Schopenhauer's will to engage in philosophy and write his essays to change the course of his life. We will also see how Schopenhauer places the Western and Eastern worlds in apparent conflict. However, in the way of the Tao, the true goal to be pursued is the realization of the Self, which is what the people whose biographies we have written about have accomplished.

10.1.3.1 The Text and the Context

The text is us, human beings, the context, the environment around us. Leonardo da Vinci father's, the context, observed his son's drawings, and immediately understood his talent and sent him to study painting in Verrocchio's workshop. The text is Coco Chanel, who knew how to sew and thus was able to create her first dresses; the context is Etienne de Balsan, her lover, who financed her first small boutique in Paris. The text is Jane Austin, and the context is a family to whom she read her narratives to in the evenings around by the fireside and who invited her to continue writing. The text was Luis Pasteur, and the context is the faculty dean who sensed the researcher's genius and sent him to the Ecole Normale Superior. The text was

Vincent Van Gogh, with his talent, and his love for painting and nature; the context of his brother Theo, who pays for his canvases, paints and brushes.

The geniuses, however, were not without their challenges. Some aspects of Van Gogh's social context were, mostly had a great bond with his brother to look forward to. Here, then, are the "losers" in life who will be successful in a fertile context after their death. Tesla and Semmelweiss, despite having proven to be great researchers, seem to fall short in intrapersonal and interpersonal intelligence due to their aggressiveness, (perhaps stems from lack of recognition) and are not accepted by the scientific community consequently.

For Semmelweiss, his end was even darker because the asylum awaited him, having been considered insane. Asylums in those days were places towards an early and agonizing death as a result of torture, cold showers, straitjackets, and beatings, from which he may have died. The ritual of hand-washing that Semmelweiss left us with was well known from ancient times in classical, pagan religious systems; the Greeks had a deity for hygiene, Hygeia; in the Talmud, it is recorded that one must wash one's hands on many occasions including after touching the corpse and returning from Cemeteries, as well as in the Quran, the theme of personal hygiene is very much present. To acknowledge Semmelweis as the one who taught us to wash our hands everywhere is something of a distortion because religious knowledge had foreseen the goodness of the hygienic rule for millennia. Nonetheless, Dr. Semmelweiss taught us to wash our hands in the clinical context, where the "infectious material" from corpses was brought into contact with women in labour. The medical and scientific context was blind to Semmelweis's intuition since behind this concept was the implied belief in a "dirty doctor" and probably antagonistic to religious doctrine, as it could have been perceived as a superstition. Semmelweiss's Voluntas was to save the human lives of disadvantaged women, but due to the violence of the medical establishment, lacking emotional intelligence, was inappropriately handled.

The text was Emily Dickinson, the context the publishers who had told her that the poems she wrote were outside the aesthetic canons of the time. Her Room, a seemingly sacred space, was a shelter to conceal her illness and against the context so acerbic and hostile to her thoughts. Only her sister, another part of the context, acknowledged her poetry once Emily died and took it upon herself to ensure the publication of her sister's manuscripts.

10.1.4 Recognition

By "recognition," also commonly names as "acknowledgment," I mean the first family members, teachers, and neighbours who recognize one's talent and inclination, not boundless success. Without this first contextual recognition, necessary to channel one's inclinations, the activity of genius cannot exist.

Access to our most authentic identity sometimes occurs not only through intuitive introspection, as Paul Ricoeur" [3] philosopher of the Art of Recognition, tells us, but through a more extended diversion involving language, the ability to act, and the emergence of moral responsibility. The Self, an accusative and reflexive pronoun, accesses its own identity through the Other he/she encounters, thus only by understanding oneself as other are our acts/works able to flourish—through an indirect manifestation of his/her identity. It is more complex to understand what we can excel at; Ricoeur says that the encounter with the Other helps us understand our meaning in the world.

The brilliant people met in these lines have all been recognized, in life or after death, but how many geniuses have remained in obscurity because the context did not recognize them out of an inability to understand their value?

This lack of mutual respect and recognition is a sort of robbery, a denial instigated by violence and unhappiness. The world of adults, parents, family members, and teachers want (even if we think they must) to sense and identify the talents of their children, grandchildren, and pupils in order to recognize their talents and direct them towards choices that enhance them, and not projective desires that are not sufficiently understood by "seniors."

By analogy, we would love to see a healthcare ecosystem where doctors can recognize, as Rita Charon writes in her definition of Narrative Medicine, their patients through intersubjectivity, the best drug to build affiliation and trust towards a more peaceful and effective system [4].

10.1.5 Smart Healthcare Providers

Through analogies we can apply the multiple intelligences we read about earlier to everyday clinical practice in the health care system.

We know that in some cases, the time allowed for a doctor to visit a patient is 10 min: intuition, beyond cognitive logic and mathematical intelligence based on statistics, remains a handy form of intelligence given such a short time [5]. Visual-spatial intelligence is that which allows one to appreciate the body language of the patient, musical intelligence produces an attention to tone of the voice. Intrapersonal intelligence is reflecting on questions such as, "what emotions and thoughts does this person evoke in me? Can I feel the proper empathy, or is there something that attracts or bothers me"? Only after looking inside, perhaps through written reflection, as Rita Charon teaches us in the use of a parallel chart, after having considered possible projections and prejudices towards the patient, will we be able to open the space for interpersonal intelligence, the kind that promotes peace, trust with assertiveness, and mitigates conflict and mistrust.

And how can I grow in bodily-kinesthetic intelligence, alongside my patient(s)? Maybe I smile, hold his/her hand, get closer to better listen, or take one step back since something annoys me, as I prefer to take some time to look inside myself before giving a cheap answer.

There is also a moral intelligence to consider. Someone with high moral intelligence may ask themselves questions like, "Am I applying the right therapy, the one also desired by the patient, or am I imposing myself through excessive medicalization? And is therapeutic obstinacy, in a sense, the negation of natural intelligence?"

Someone with an understanding of nature is familiar with the seasons of a person's life, there is a time for birthing, and an end; a time to work and a time to rest.

Furthermore, one with existential intelligence asks, "What is this patient talking to me about, apart from the physical pains in the body and the abnormalities in the lab tests or scans? *Sic stantibus rebus,* i.e., apart from the fact that there is illness, what are the life aspirations of the individual in front of me?" [6].

Am I alone in all this, or through the interpersonal and moral intelligence of the group? Is it possible to create a harmonic care team comprising, composing metaphorically beautiful music, a constellation not only of doctors but also of nurses, social workers, volunteers, and family members, so as not to leave the patient and all too often his or her family alone?

On the language we use, can we make ourselves better understood, to make an impact with linguistic intelligence, with the beauty and aesthetics of a sentence bordering on poetry that can touch the mind and heart of the listener?

However, above all, can we take pleasure in caring and curing for others, loving the job, and cultivating it with playfulness, light years far removed from sadistic humour and cynical banter that keeps burnout and compassion away?

Can we still marvel at the experience of each patient's story, written or spoken. What about the narratives of colleagues, understanding that they are essential nourishment for profession growth?

Water that irrigates a parched soil, where one can plant seeds whose shoots we will see? That is the *Voluntas,* the willingness driven by *eros*-type love (romantic love) that leads all the Brilliant Masters we have mentioned to innovate, discover, live, express themselves, and play an active role in this world.

Yes, of course, all the qualities we mentioned cannot be equally developed in a single individual. The geniuses examined, from Dante to Dickinson, from the Beatles to Beth Harmon, possessed different combinations of these intelligences and to different degrees. However, they all had inner strength and the potential to pursue what they wished to be, which coincided with doing.

Not belonging to the mainstream school of thought of the last century, that of evidence-based medicine, or rather knowing how to belong to it without giving up the other intellectual possibilities related to the world of intuition, expressiveness, and artistic gestures, means broadening the options to become a constantly evolving health professional, and therefore, points of reference for one's patients. It means, increasing in self-awareness to reap more peace with oneself and the world around him.

The reasons for dissatisfaction amongst healthcare workers stems from a perception of time that never passes, a perceived meaninglessness in the daily activities performed, the mere waiting for the month-end salary, the obsessive planning of vacation time, the disinterest in the proposed education, and the loss of respect and trust for one's colleagues and patients.

The good news is that we now realize how important it is to be serene and at peace, and to have find purpose for our careers. COVID-19 has been a detonator to exposing faulty decisions, as well as correct ones. We have heard from so many doctors and nurses who, although traumatized by the unprecedented amount of death, are happy and proud that they were able to be there to help, as a mission, their self-realization.

Innovative doctors and healthcare workers can make choices of that harvest happiness and eudaimonia rather than those that are prompted by selfish ambition (as Schopenhauer fought against). What good is it to work tirelessly, and not enjoy the fruits of your labour? In Dante's last triplet in the paradise of his Divine Comedy he writes, "Amor che move il Sole e l'altre Stelle...," which translates to, "the Love that moves the sun and the other stars..."

> 'Who in the world am I?' Ah, that is the great puzzle!
> Lewis Carroll, Alice in Wonderland

10.1.6 Healthcare Wonderland

I wish to begin this last section pf the book with the Italian word "Meraviglia," or rather from the Latin word *mirabilia*, meaning "admirable things," also from the verb *mirari*, "to look with wonder." This word describes the experience of being filled with admiration and awe at new things, at the extraordinary, at the phenomena of nature, "the sublime," Kant called it, "the starry sky above me," and at the unknown. Moreover, the Latin word is probably the result of a blending of the words "mir-abilia" arising from the prefix mir-, "to look" and *habilis*, "capable of," things capable of being looked at. We are thus in visual perception, remembering that for the Greeks and Latins, "looking" was also knowing.

In English, the meaning of the word "Wonder" is connected to the meaning of the word "Wander." Alice goes to Wonderland (as we studied in Chap. 8), with a play on words, as usual, polysemic since Lewis Carroll plays with words; she goes to the world of Wanderers to figure out who she is in the world, and she hears the riddle "'Who in the world am I?' Ah, that is the great puzzle!"

Wonder is, for English-speakers, something that is not only related to the sense of seeing but to our movements; the word connotes a sense of being lost, distracted, or a lack of concentration. Furthermore, to generate *wonder*, the invitation is to leave the best-known paths (maybe the EBM-cracy, the possible violence of the establishment, the terrible workload) and embrace the unknown paths, an inner journey which we simply do not know.

To wonder means to change the mindset, moving from a *Vita Activa* to rediscovering the art of lingering; in the *Vita Contemplativa* as Byung–Chul Han, a Korean Philosopher who advocated for doing less, which when applied to a healthcare context means less talking, less prescribing, less medicalizing, but more listening to, more seeing, being more present and focused as in contemplation [7].

Thus, our possible daily masterpiece in this wandering in "Healthcare Wonderland" is to get up every morning with a good reason to celebrate our Non-Birthday as The Mad Hatter does at the Tea Party in which Alice participates. A wonderfully simple reason. To celebrate every day of life as carers of ourselves and others.

10.2 Practice Time of This Last Chapter

10.2.1 *The Listening Scale*

In Narrative Medicine, a few types of keys to interpreting the narratives between health professionals and patients are preponderant: the most universal is that of Arthur Kleimann [8], who distinguished how the health/pathology pair is talked about into the categories of Disease (a mechanical triggering cause). Illness (living with illness and its repercussions on daily life) and Sickness (the social inclusion or exclusion of the sick person).

Another well-established reading key is Arthur Frank's, which confronts us with how we cope with the course of an illness: "Chaos," where there is no awareness of the experience by the patient; "Restitution," adherence to therapy is maximised in anticipation of having health as a reward; and "Quest," which means what patient learns from the illness and what new lifestyles she/he can adopt, compatible with the loss of function of body and mind [9].

There are so many other possible keys to aid in the interpretation of narratives like that of Mike Bury, who goes to identify trends in moral judgment in narratives of physicians, patients, and caregivers. From his findings he invents the word "faction," a conjunction of the words "fact" and "fiction" to describe how a narrative can be filled with truths and fictional details at the same time [10]. Another example is Robert Plutchick [11], who focuses on the analyses of emotions that emerge in narratives. Lastly, Jonathan Launer, who seeks to understand the dynamism of the narrative, assumes that a static story is problematic in that it is indicative of a relationship between caregiver and cared for that does not evolve.

The thing that is reported most by patients is whether the health professional listened to the person, whether they are allowed to speak, and whether they felt they had a choice in their treatment. From studies published in the literature, it is known that the healthcare professional talks much more than he or she listens (more *vita activa* than *vita contemplativa*), often failing to show curiosity about the person, which is the basis of care. Also, patients who "inhabit" their bodies, know them, and beyond their bodies, know their desires for how to live their lives. The health professionals most loved by patients and those in whom people place their utmost trust are those who are not only very knowledgeable demonstrate a capacity to listen to the patient's wishes. They allow the right time for processing information, not only for the person seeking treatment, but also for themselves. In this way, they have more time to come to a shared decisions about a recovery plan. Patients are not the only one who need to reflect, but the physician also needs time to determine if he or she fully understands their patient more than just what is written about them in a micro section of clinical history.

I'm deeply grateful to the anaesthesiologist Giorgio Bardellini, with whom we have developed a possible checklist to evaluate how reciprocal listening was during a doctor's visit.

Dr. Bardellini suggested that at the end of a Narrative Clinical Visit, or a pathway in which the patient followed narratively as well; one can collect both voices of those who were actors in the pathway (or more than two voices) through a minimum semi-structured double interview to be distributed to patients, which includes the following fields:

For the physician or other health professional:
Age of physician ...Gender...
Social status...
Age of patient...Gender...Social status...
Disease...Onset...Other considerations...

1. Did I listen to the patient? From 1 (not at all) to 7 (completely)
2. Did I interrupt the patient? From 1 (not at all) to 7 (completely)
3. Did the patient interrupt me? From 1 (not at all) to 7 (completely)
4. Did the patient talk to me about the disease? From 1 (not at all) to 7 (completely)
5. Did I talk about the disease? From 1 (not at all) to 7 (completely)
6. Did the patient tell me about her/his life plans? From 1 (not at all) to 7 (completely)
7. Did I talk about the patient's life plans? From 1 (not at all) to 7 (completely)
8. Did I feel the need to impose myself? From 1 (not at all) to 7 (completely)
9. Did the patient impose herself/himself? From 1 (not at all) to 7 (completely)
10. Did we make some decisions together? From 1 (not at all) to 7 (completely)
11. Overall, did we talk to each other, listen to each other, and understand other? From 1 (not at all) to 7 (completely)
12. How did I feel during the visit/visits? From 1(very bad) to 7 (very good)

Comment on the moments of interruption, imposition and shared decision-making..

For the Patient:
Age of patient...Gender...Social status...
Disease...onset...Other considerations...

1. Did I listen to the carer (physician or other care professional)? From 1 (not at all) to 7 (completely)
2. Did I interrupt the carer? From 1 (not at all) to 7 (completely)
3. Did the carer interrupt me? From 1 (not at all) to 7 (completely)
4. Did the carer tell me about the disease? From 1 (not at all) to 7 (completely)
5. Did I talk about my illness? From 1 (not at all) to 7 (completely)
6. Did I talk about my life plans? From 1 (not at all) to 7 (completely)
7. Did the carer tell me about my life plans? From 1 (not at all) to 7 (completely)
8. Did I have to impose myself? From 1 (not at all) to 7 (completely)
9. Did the carer seem to impose herself/himself? From 1 (not at all) to 7 (completely)

10. Did we make some decisions together? From 1 (not at all) to 7 (completely)
11. Overall, did we talk to each other, listen to each other, and understand each other? From 1 (not at all) to 7 (completely)
12. How did I feel during the visit/visits? From 1(very bad) to 7 (very good)

Comment on the moments of interruption, imposition and shared decision-making...

This brief interview can be conducted over a chosen period, and after acquiring the necessary informed consent signatures.

Beginning to apply a listening assessment, dividing the time when talking about illness from when talking about life plans can be a first simple tool to understand the usefulness of listening to the clinical history and the biography contextualized to the patient's health status.

Numbers and metrics can sometimes be very useful when applied to "narrative skills" and not only to EBM. Creativity is also the skill of finding effective measures for what is deemed impossible or too vague to be worthy of a metric.

Short notice to explain the scale: Interruption, imposition, and lack of shared decision-making are small acts of violence. Liberty to choose not to follow the medical prescription is granted. Liberty not to insult and lack of respect towards the doctor is an act of violence. The listening tool should accurately allow a pacifistic rhythm of conversation among doctors and patients. This metric could also be adapted among colleagues to evaluate the climate of the work culture, like a thermometer.

Now we will move on from the disease and the illness of the patient into the realm of the existential, their demonstrated willingness (Voluntas). We will practice listening to broaden our horizons and tease out the deep wishes of the person before us.

10.2.2 Nesting Multiple Intelligence with Not Violent Communication

1. Visionary geniuses, multiple intelligences and talents

    It would be interesting to investigate by which mentioned geniuses you felt drawn to, as well as some other brilliant, outstanding, geniuses not contemplated in the lines before. Let this be an indication of an archetypal model chosen to admire and to imitate. Two other possible figures could be Alain Turing, the mathematician who decoded the Nazi code during the second world war, or Florence Nightingale, the woman who revolutionized Victorian hospitals, bringing clean air and lines, windows, and more nourishing food to the structures. Or both?

    Then, explore the beauty of our multiple intelligence (effortless but precious online questionnaires might give us some suggestions). Please find the link to the test developed by Howard Gardner. https://www.idrlabs.com/multiple-intelligences/test.php. Once you've got the result, you can decide whether to invest in equalizing them or investing in those you love most.

After this, contemplate your talents, those driven by your willingness, in your personal and professional biography, and see if there are roads not taken that you would like to travel.
2. Non-violent communication and multiple intelligence

Non-violent communication is synonymous with winning peaceful situations.

We have seen the four steps of violent communication: Observations/fact-checking, Feelings, Needs and Requests. Multiple intelligences apply to each step of this process.

> **Observation**: *Visual-spatial intelligence, Natural Intelligence, Musical Intelligence, Fast Cognitive Intelligence (intuition).*
> **Feelings**: *Intrapersonal Intelligence and Interpersonal Intelligence, bodily intelligence.*
> **Needs**: *Existential intelligence, moral intelligence, body intelligence, reflective cognitive intelligence, mathematical intelligence (dimensional intelligence).*
> **Request**: *Linguistic intelligence (narrative intelligence).*

The frame above is the first attempt to link the multiple intelligences to the four steps of non-violent communication we have learned in this book. So, you, reader, are free to change it and try it during your peaceful visit or to de-escalate conflicts with colleagues' patients, in public communication at scientific congresses or with the citizenship group.
3. An application of multiple intelligences in narrative medicine research: The prader-will. Syndrome Study [12]. Why only rely on the IQ to evaluate intelligence?

Prader-Willi syndrome (PWS) significantly impacts health-related quality of life; however, its relational and existential aspects remain unknown in Italian clinical and social debate. The project aimed to investigate the impact of PWS on illness experience through Narrative Medicine (NM) to understand the daily life, needs and resources of patients with PWS and their caregivers and to furnish insights for clinical practice. Unfortunately, these people are often called derogatory slurs.

The project involved ten medical centres of the Italian Network for Rare Diseases and PWS family associations and targeted underage and adult patients with PWS and their caregivers. Written interviews, composed of a sociodemographic survey and a narrative component, were collected through the project's website. Three dedicated illness plots employed evocative and open statements to facilitate individual expression and to encourage reflection. Narratives were analysed using NVivo software. Researchers discussed the results with the project's steering committee.

Twenty-one children and adolescents, and 34 adults with PWS joined the project, as well as 138 caregivers. A PWS diagnosis or the caregiving of a patient with PWS older than five years was the eligibility criteria, as well as the willingness to share their illness experience by writing and the ability to communicate in Italian. The analysis of narratives led to understanding the PWS social and relational issues concerning diagnosis and current management, PWS daily experiences and social contexts, PWS implications in a work context, and participants' perspectives on the future. Narratives demonstrated that PWS management affects relationships and work-life balance, and that social stigma remains.

The project represented the first effort to investigate the impact of PWS on social experiences in Italy through NM while considering the perspectives of patients with PWS and their caregivers. The findings indicated that a multi-professional approach is fundamental to ensure adequate treatment and provide elements for its improvement.

Talking about PWS emerged as a taboo. In illness-centred and sickness-centred narratives, 28 caregivers encountered significant difficulties in socializing the challenges that PWS imposes on daily life, as well as the pain of having a child that is "different." We identify this as a "social pain" that concerns caregivers when performing familiar criticalities. Furthermore, caregivers considered the project a chance to invite society to integrate people with PWS and to denounce the stigma that surrounds them. If the literature demonstrates cognitive impairment in people with PWS, we would like to enrich the evidence by suggesting the consideration of the multiple intelligences these people demonstrate in their everyday experiences. In line with Gardner's reflection, revealing alternatives to the standard forms of intelligence (the logical-mathematical and linguistic ones), the people with Prader-Willi narratives demonstrated the constant use of visual-spatial, musical, interpersonal, existential and introspective talents, resources and capabilities. In this regard, individuals with PWS have been reported to show above-average performance in several tasks, implying visual-spatial skills, which are linked with higher math abilities in the general population. In particular, the importance of multiple intelligences emerged in food-control strategies and activities, suggesting that considering them may positively influence the overall illness experience.

What do you think about applying multiple intelligence frameworks to your current clinical or social services? How about in research? Please take the time to reflect upon it. They could be extremely useful in health promotion and well-being, and in fighting the stigma around physical and mental conditions. Would you like to write about it?

10.2.3 Moving from Violence to Peace

4. Peace

We have been speaking about violence and its etymological roots, but what about peace and its building elements?

Peace comes from the Anglo-French *pes* and means "freedom from civil disorder" and *pais* "reconciliation," "silence," "permission." The Latin word *Pax* has a different flavour: "compact," "agreement," "treaty," "tranquility." From Pax comes the word PACT, a "binding together" [13].

The ancient roots are Indo-European, related to *pag-* and *pak*, to" bind" and to "pay," very rational and pragmatic words.

In Greek mythology, Peace (*Eirene*) is a goddess associated with the spring season, which ensures the prosperity of the land and people, abundant food, and harmony. Peace, along with her two sisters *Eunomia* (Good Law) and *Dike* (Justice), is guardian of the gates of Olympus and administers wealth for humanity.

The Greek poet Hesiod, in his "Works and Days," left us with the effect of *Eirene*, together with her two sisters [14]:

But for those who make straightforward judgments is, those who invoke the goddess Dike (justice)-to strangers and men of the land, and do not depart from what is right, the city prospers, and the people thrive in it: Eirene (Peace), the nurturer of the children, is a stranger in their land, and all-seeing Zeus never decrees a cruel war against them. Neither famine nor disaster ever haunts the men who do true justice (Dike), but lightly, they take care of the fields with all their attention. The land there brings abundant provisions; on the mountains, the oak brings acorns on top and bees in between. Their woolly sheep are laden with fleece; their women bear children like their parents. They bloom good things continually, and they do not have to travel by ship, for the land that gives grain bears them fruit.

Nevertheless, are there specific studies to investigate the key elements of peace, which are its pillars? Yes, and somehow, the family described in the ancient myth mirrors the elements.

The measurement of peace was proposed based on these qualities: Emotional Tone, Agency, Hope, Tolerance, Basic Needs, Safety, and Group Cohesion [15]. They are all positively interrelated: if Basic Needs are not satisfied—i.e. the famine described by Hesiod-then peace may waver. If *Polemos* (the Greek word for war) outbreaks in the group's cohesion, then Peace wavers.

Beyond the results indicating the level of peace in the community, I find it remarkable to focus on its elements and to discover that they belong to the multidimensional model of health and well-being. By now we should know them very well: authentic self-expression which incorporates our talents and creates a sense of agency, tolerance (that today we could also add resilience), learning to effectively regulate our Emotions, and Hope, not merely rational optimism, but the kind that is founded on Faith, Grace and Contemplation.

If you wish now, consider the fundamental elements for peacebuilding in your professional life, your organization, your multidisciplinary equipment, and your patients and their caregivers.

In 2020, the World Health Organization issued the guidelines entitled Health and Peace [16]:

WHO will deliver aid by humanitarian principles (of humanity, neutrality, impartiality, and operational independence) and international humanitarian law. It is precisely because of the need to uphold humanitarian principles and to "do no harm" that health workers are required to have a robust understanding of the dynamics and drivers of conflict and the root causes of social unrest. This awareness allows humanitarian action to be designed in a conflict-sensitive manner.

However, WHO does not include only people in war countries, but promotes also "*micro-peace*" (I invented this neologism, hoping it can convey peace in the tiniest situations and things)) within the communities through trust building and reciprocal dialogue.

Peace has always been this illustrious good sought after throughout history. We need it to operate in a healthier healthcare system for both current and future generations. This is why we cannot settle down, but we must learn and commit to taking our daily dose of smartness and geniality.

The vulnerable Emily Dickinson writes,
I many times thought peace had come
When peace was far away—
As Wrecked Men—deem they sight the land—
At the Centre of the Sea—
And struggle slacker—but to prove
As hopelessly as I—
How many of the fictitious Shores—
Before the Harbor be—

Let's build this harbour for Emily, the fragile and vulnerable people, but primarily for ourselves.

In the following last lines, we will review the results of a narrative Italian survey carried out by ISTUD for the Health Ministry on young students with the topic of sport, health promotion, and doping [17]. The students were asked to write about the concept *of winning or losing*: 74 students participated, mean age 17, 40% boys, 58% girls, and 2% did not specify.

The narratives of some students reveal that winning for me is…*"Very Important; in fact, I see defeat as a total failure,"* but also *"unnecessary if you do something with passion."* For someone else, winning is just *"[…] for me, having set a goal and having achieved it."*

When asked about losing, the teenagers emerge from the frequent use of the words *"Important, a lesson to be learned, a path, normal, fundamental, teaching…"; "Normal to lose, to fail is normal, it is part of our life's path, and we must accept losing failure when it happens to us to become stronger and push ourselves even harder."*

They write about the importance of losing. Notice the formulation of a wise hero, even when beaten, in their words. This feature shows an uncommon maturity and an ability to process even the unpleasant events that life holds in store. They are not frightened by it; their reflexivity about competition is admirable.

Lastly, their consideration about doping: *"It is a consequence of society's pressure on athletes. We should accept that we are human, sometimes less strong than other humans."* A common and shared idea is that it is highly wrong and unfair that students have doping substances from the perspective of more healthy and balanced competition. *"I think doping is playing with an advantage at the cost of risking your health; we can compete cleanly and healthily without the need for other substances; you just have to train to achieve a fair goal."*

Wonder. Awe. This is what I feel reading their narratives.

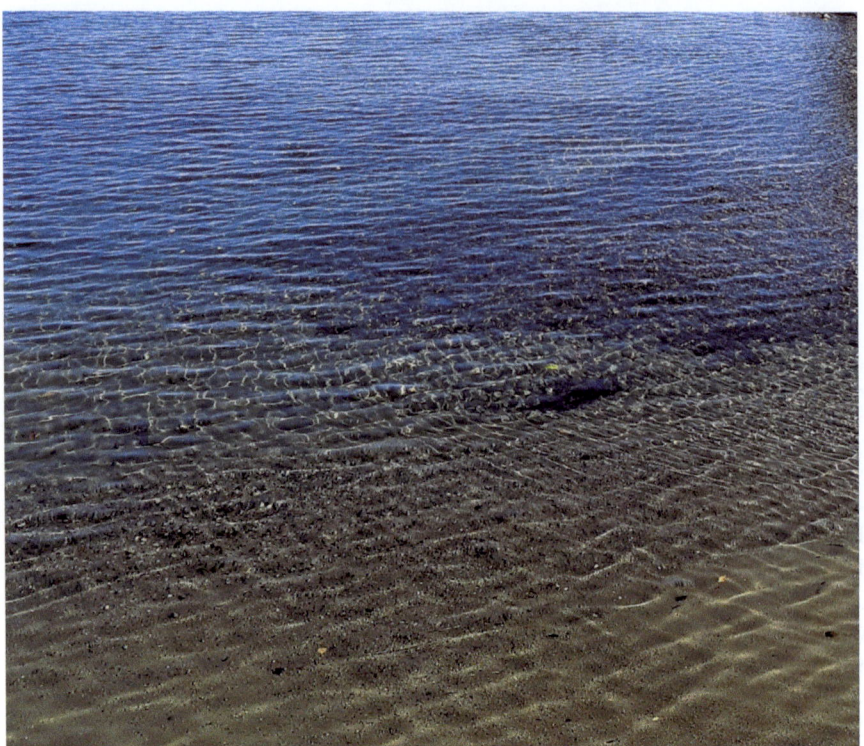

Fig. 10.1 *Transparent words (phot by Maria Giulia Marini)*

Let's achieve fair goals, promoting well-being and health in a clean, peaceful, not over competitive and harmful way: this is what our children are teaching us (Fig. 10.1).

References

1. https://www.medicinanarrativa.eu/consigli-per-essere-geniali; 2021.
2. Gardner, Howard, Multiple intelligences: new horizons in theory and practice" New Horizon, 2006.
3. Ricoeur P. Oneself as another. University of Chicago Press; 1995.
4. Charon R. Narrative medicin: honoring the stories of illness. Oxford University Press; 2006.
5. Launer J. How not to be a Doctor: and other essays. CRC Press; 2007.
6. Gavin F. Recovery: the lost art of convalescence. Wellcome Collection; 2022.
7. Han, Byung-Chul. The scent of time: a philosophical essay on the art of lingering, 1st Polity, 2017.
8. Kleinmann, Arthur. The illness narrative, suffering, healing and the human condition". Academic Medicine (2017).
9. Frank A. Th wounded storyteller. 2nd. University of Chicago Press; 2013.
10. Bury M. Illness narratives: fact or fiction? Sociol Health Illness. 2001;23(3):263–85.

11. Slama ME, Plutchik R. Emotions and life: perspectives from psychology, biology, and evolution. Psychology and Marketing (s.d.). 2000.
12. Ragusa L, et al. Caring and living with Prader-Willi syndrome in Italy: integrating children, adults and parents' experiences through a multicenter narrative medicine research. BMJ Open. 2020;10(8):e036502.
13. https://www.etymonline.com/word/pax
14. Hesiod. Work and days. 700 BC. https://chs.harvard.edu/primary-source/hesiod-works-and-days-sb/
15. Zucker H, et al. Development of a scale to measure individuals' ratings of peace. Confl Heal. 2016;
16. WHO. Health and peace. 2020. https://www.who.int/initiatives/who-health-and-peace-initiative
17. Quotidiano sanità. Doping, sport e disabilità fisica. 2023.

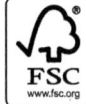

MIX
Papier aus verantwortungsvollen Quellen
Paper from responsible sources
FSC® C105338

If you have any concerns about our products,
you can contact us on
ProductSafety@springernature.com

In case Publisher is established outside the EU,
the EU authorized representative is:
**Springer Nature Customer Service Center GmbH
Europaplatz 3, 69115 Heidelberg, Germany**

Printed by Libri Plureos GmbH
in Hamburg, Germany